The Insiders' Guide
To Medical Schools
2004/2005

Published by Blackwell Publishing Ltd
Blackwell Publishing, Inc., 350 Main Street, Malden, Massachusetts 02148-5020, USA
Blackwell Publishing Ltd, 9600 Garsington Road, Oxford OX4 2DQ, UK
Blackwell Publishing Asia Pty Ltd, 550 Swanston Street, Carlton, Victoria 3053, Australia

First published 1998
Second Edition 1999
Third Edition 2000
Fourth Edition 2001
Fifth Edition 2002
Reprinted 2002
Sixth Edition 2003
Reprinted 2003
Seventh Edition 2004

W 19

A050281

ISBN 0-7279-1851-6

Catalogue records for this title are available from the British Library and the Library of Congress

Set in India by Siva Math Setters, Chennai
Printed and bound in the Spain by GraphyCems

Commissioning Editor: Mary Banks
Development Editor: Nic Ulyatt
Production Controller: Kate Charman

Cartoons © Clive Featherstone

For further information on Blackwell Publishing, visit our website:
http://www.blackwellpublishing.com

The publisher's policy is to use permanent paper from mills that operate a sustainable forestry policy, and
which has been manufactured from pulp processed using acid-free and elementary chlorine-free practices.
Furthermore, the publisher ensures that the text paper and cover board used have met acceptable
environmental accreditation standards.

Contents

Jennie Ciechan is in her final year of medicine at Edinburgh University. Having chaired the UK Medical Students Committee for the last 2 years, Jennie is enjoying a return to a more active social life.

Sally Girgis is Secretary of the Medical Students Committee at the British Medical Association. She is an Australian who has lived in London for the past four years.

Philip Smith is a year 5 medical student at the University of Nottingham. He is from 'Up North' and proud of it! He plans to live life to the full and to enjoy a long and successful career.

Foreword

"When a dream takes hold of you…run with it."

Patch Adams

If you are reading this you are considering a career in medicine, a profession that existed before universities and colleges, or even the word "medicine" itself. As human beings we have always been curious about the human body and have desired to help the physical and mental needs of those around us, whether we realised it or not. The study and practise of medicine gives a unique and trusted insight into the lives of people who need some form of assistance. People will share very personal information with their doctor, some of which even their nearest and dearest may not be aware of. Communication skills and integrity, as well as the development of scientific knowledge, are the groundings that you must obtain in all medical courses.

The study of medicine is constantly evolving, and the advancements are so rapid that your university education can only be considered a foundation block for life-long learning; an invaluable skill in all walks of life. On the road to becoming a doctor, you will be met with uncertainty, ethical dilemmas, and emotional challenges. Thirty years down the line things will still surprise you, and patients will still rely upon you. It is these privileges that make such a vocation a great one, and one of which you can be proud.

On this note, it is essential that you choose a university that will allow you to flourish, that will offer challenge and excitement, as well as an educational environment that suits your personal learning needs. Medical education, like clinical medicine, undergoes constant change to ensure that it caters for the growing volume of students. For a long time the UK Medical Students Committee has been campaigning for wider participation in medical schools and the last decade has seen the demography of the medical student body change. On commencing your studies you will encounter other school leavers, graduates, nurses, lawyers, and journalists who all add to the diversity of the student body. Although these changes have been warmly welcomed, more needs to be done to attract students from less affluent backgrounds.

On choosing a university you must also ask, 'What can I offer in return?' If you are passionate about something, check the university websites to ensure that they cater for your extracurricular requirements. If you are a professional sailor, Plymouth may be an ideal destination. If it is rugby, Scotland is the obvious application ground; we need fresh blood in the team! Ultimately the path to becoming a doctor is more than just sitting in anatomy and biochemistry lectures, essential as these are. University is a unique period in life where principles and beliefs can be challenged, mistakes made, and lessons learned. It is a time where you can refine your dreams and expectations, then start the journey towards making them a reality. If medicine is one of these dreams, I am positive that you will not be disappointed with the future that is awaiting you at your chosen university.

Foreword

This book provides an outline of the experience offered at all UK medical schools, and is produced by the British Medical Association's Medical Students Committee (MSC). The Editors and other contributors have worked extremely hard to produce a balanced and well informed publication. I hope it will empower you with the information to choose the most suitable course.

On behalf of the committee, good luck with your application.

Leigh Bissett
Chairman
BMA Medical Students Committee

Preface

"The life so short, the craft so long to learn"

Hippocrates on medicine

Choosing to study medicine is a great undertaking. To the majority it is still considered more than a job, rather a vocation – a way of life. It will challenge you mentally, physically, emotionally, and financially. Despite the heavy workload and increasing cost of studying medicine, medics, as doctors in training, enjoy a very privileged position. We are given the opportunity to work with our patients during some of their most difficult and personal moments, and our course is a unique blend of science and humanities. On completion of the undergraduate course, we have the ability to enter into a phenomenally worthwhile and rewarding career in which our primary objective must be to serve. Doctors are some of the most trusted professionals across the world, respected by all ethnic, religious, and cultural groups. This is why a degree in medicine can take you anywhere and gives the opportunity to enjoy such a vast variety of experiences. Equally though, doctors carry a great burden of responsibility. They treat the most vulnerable in society and, often, individual decisions that they make influence whether a patient will survive or not.

The experiences you have at medical school will remain with you throughout your long careers. Although the common goal of qualification as a doctor is the same at all medical schools, the diverse nature of these institutions means that the training experience differs considerably depending on where you study. Therefore, if you choose to apply to medical school we feel you should have the information to make the most informed choice possible, so you can make the **best** choice possible for **you**. This right choice is not simply the decision as to whether to study medicine or not, but includes thoughts on which medical schools to apply to, what assessment structures will best suit you, and the atmosphere in which you will thrive the most.

This book is a compilation of what we feel you should know, regarding both *what studying medicine really involves* and what characterises the individual medical schools. The strength of this book lies in the fact that it has been written by students, for students, and each medical school chapter is written by a current medical student at that school; hence *The Insiders' Guide*. Their personal insight into the various institutions is an invaluable resource and provides opinions that are not always found in medical school prospectuses or in the UCAS handbook. A book like this could never claim to be totally objective or definitive about all the differences and similarities, or strengths and weaknesses between the medical schools. However, every effort has been made to ensure that the opinions of the medical students who contributed to the book are based on factual information.

Undoubtedly different people are suited to different styles of learning, and it is important that you use this book, in conjunction with the university prospectuses, to help you choose the kind of institution, course, and location that's right for you. Indeed, not everyone is suited to a career in medicine at all, and it is important that you have thought carefully about your own aspirations and dreams before you apply. Take the opportunities available to visit the medical schools that you are most interested in and speak to as many students as you can whilst you are there in order to canvass their experiences and views. Time spent carefully in consideration now will make an instrumental difference to both your enjoyment and success at medical school.

The right choice is down to the individual – everyone is different! We hope that the information in this book will help you make the most suitable choice for you. Remember: although this is a very daunting period, always maintain your enthusiasm, remain optimistic, and, most importantly of all, pursue your desires to the best of your abilities.

Good luck and best wishes for the future.

Jennie Ciechan, Sally Girgis, and Philip Smith

Acknowledgements and contributors

We would like to thank all the many individuals and institutions who have provided the information and views contained in this book. It would not have been possible without their help. We would also like to thank the numerous BMA and BMJ staff who have contributed at various stages in the preparation of this book. Their support and efforts on our behalf have been invaluable and are very much appreciated. In particular we should like to extend our warmest thanks to Christina Karaviotis (production) and Sneha Sangyam (admissions office liaison) who have worked tirelessly on the book despite very busy schedules, and to Ellie Babbington for her tireless support and morale boosting skills.

The need for an *Insiders' Guide* and the vision for its production were first dreamt up many years ago by members of the Medical Students Committee who have long since graduated and are busy working as doctors. Each edition has built upon the hard work and ideas of the editions that have preceded it and to these past pioneers and editors we are extremely grateful. Finally we would like to thank all the members of the BMA's Medical Students Committee, both past and present, who have contributed to the *Insiders' Guide*. We believe that it is a fantastic resource and we hope that it will continue to go from strength to strength in the years to come.

If you have any suggestions for ways in which the *Insiders' Guide* could be improved, we would very much like to hear them. Please email students@bma.org.uk.

Past editors
Alex Almoudaris, Simon Calvert, Deborah Cohen, Lizz Corps, Chris Ferguson, Kristian Mears, Richard Partridge, Kinesh Patel, Jill Spencer, and Ian Urmston.

Specialist area contributors
Beverley Almeida, Dan Gibbons, Ian Harwood, Jane Margetts, Parampal Tung, and Paul Sutton.

Student contributors in the 2004/2005 edition
Alex Almoudaris, Amy Athersmith, Zubir Ahmed, Jonathan Beavers, Leigh Bissett, Joanna Burgess, David Burke, Emmie Carter, Ben Clayton, Angela Davey, Sam Davies, Lucy-Jane Davis, Mary Docherty, Catherine Fletcher, Nick France, Rohin Francis, Amir Halim, Eoin Harty, Nicholas Hipkins, Sonya Hiremath, Nishamali Jayatilleke, Stephen Kinnear, Vicky Lester, Kirsty Lloyd, Huda Mahmoud, Johann Malawana, Kitty Mohan, Raymond Oliphant, Arun Prabhu, Neil Robinson, David Rogers, Balvinder Sagoo, Frances Sansbury, Nick Thomas, Sabeen Ul-Haq, and Kristen Widdowsen.

Cartoons created by
Clive Featherstone

Editorial assistance
Matthew O'Flynn, Sneha Sangyam

With apologies to any contributors we may have accidentally missed out.

Philip's personal acknowledgements
To Beverley, my Mum, Dad, and all my family. Without you, all this would not have been possible. I love you all.

Jennie's personal acknowledgements
With thanks to Dave for his patience and support, and to my parents for working so hard in order to enable me to pursue my dreams.

Meet Mikey

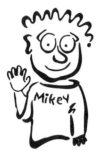

Hi, I'm Mikey.

I'm here to give you the inside information on life as a medical student and a career in medicine. To help guide you through the information in this book, it is split into two parts:

Part 1 contains insiders' information designed to help you decide whether medicine is the right choice for you, how to choose the right medical school, how to apply, and information on other important considerations such as managing your finances and dealing with hurdles.

Part 2 gives valuable information and views about every medical school in the UK, written by students at that medical school. Each medical school entry has been divided for ease into three categories: Education, Welfare, and Sports and Social. Students have also provided insight into the "great" and "bad" things about each school.

To make flicking through easier, the following symbols will appear throughout the book:

Education

Welfare

Sports and social

Great things about the medical school

Bad things about the medical school

Now, it won't surprise you that student life differs radically from one university to the next. What may surprise you is that each medical school offers a course which is to some extent unique. Medics, more than anyone else, can give you the low-down on the distinguishing features that you may want to consider. However, it is best also to make use of the other resources available, such as the university prospectuses and open day visits.

REMEMBER:

☑ Read the medical school/university prospectus.
☑ Read the alternative prospectus.
☑ Visit the medical school (most have open days) and the town or city.
☑ Talk to students studying at the medical school.
☑ Visit the medical school website.

GOOD LUCK!

A book like this could never claim to be totally objective or definitive about all the differences and similarities, or strengths and weaknesses between the medical schools. Every effort has been made to ensure that the opinions of the medical students who contributed to the book are based on factual information. Take the opinions offered here into account and we strongly recommend you use this information alongside other material you will have collected (for example, prospectuses or the opinions of others) as you draw up your shortlist of where to apply.

Part 1
Insiders' information

1

Is medicine for you?

"Some patients, though conscious that their condition is perilous, recover their health simply through their contentment with the goodness of the physician."

Hippocrates 460–400 BC

Ask the average student why they are applying to study medicine and they'll probably tell you it's because they enjoy science and want to help people. Probe a little deeper and they may mention ideas such as money, and the fact that they are expected to get good A-level grades. Medicine may even command a certain amount of kudos and possibly sex appeal!

Although trends may be changing, doctors have traditionally been held in high regard by the general public, which many students find an appealing prospect. Indeed a 2004 MORI public opinion poll reported that doctors were the most trusted profession. However, with this respect comes responsibility and pressure: one only has to read a small selection of newspapers to see that doctors are a major focus of media attention and public interest, and not all of the resulting coverage is favourable or fair.

Knowing that you are under constant scrutiny, and not always from people who understand clinical medicine, adds to the demands of the job. As a doctor you will be faced with difficult decisions involving ethical and clinical dilemmas, and these situations can be very stressful. There are also many unpleasant tasks, like breaking bad news or dealing with abusive patients or relatives, and at times you will be frustrated by the lack of resources and time available to you. Curing patients is fulfilling and exciting – it happens regularly in some specialties – but there will be many patients whom you cannot cure, many symptoms that cannot be controlled, and many "worried well" who cannot be persuaded that they are not in fact ill.

The number of people applying to study medicine continues to rise. This is partly due to the expansion of the number of medical schools and medical school places in the last few years and partly due to the increasing availability of places for applicants from non-traditional routes and for graduates on fast-track courses. However, despite the increasing number of places, there is still a shortage of doctors in the UK, which means there are more than enough jobs to go round.

Salaries for junior doctors have increased significantly over the last few years and are set to continue rising. Indeed some junior doctors can be paid an annual salary of around £34,000 before tax. It must be remembered that the workload can be very demanding and salaries reflect the working pattern, intensity of work, and the antisocial nature of the post. As you become more senior in your chosen field, pay improves, often with the scope for private income. Yet if your only aim in medicine is to make endless amounts of money, to prance around in a white coat looking like a star from a television drama, or to prove how able you are to pass exams, forget it. There are many easier ways to make money and the work is only occasionally glamorous. Application and dedication to patient care and learning are far more important attributes and a doctor's focus must be on a desire to serve. It is also worth bearing in mind that graduates from other shorter courses may be in a job and earning more money than you will be when you qualify, when you still have two more years of unpaid study left to go.

To follow particular career directions in medicine you will need to study hard and sit a number of postgraduate exams after qualifying. It is vital that you continue your medical education if you are to keep your skills and knowledge up to date and, even as a consultant, you will be required to regularly prove your expertise and grasp of current developments. It's a long haul, and requires a commitment and devotion that far exceed any financial rewards. Whilst many of your friends in other professions will be able to relax at the end of a working day, you may finish a long shift only to have to begin your study for the evening, and young doctors frequently spend their weekends working. Whatever combination of reasons has made you consider medicine, remember it is a vocation. Those who enter medical school with a strong commitment to work hard, learn, and serve patients to their best ability are the people most likely to find life as a doctor richly rewarding and stimulating.

The medical profession is increasingly diverse, with ethnic minorities comprising 30% of the intake to medical school and women approximately 60%. It would be untrue to say that racial and sexual discrimination does not occur in medical schools or the health service, but the BMA, NHS Executive, and all medical schools are active in promoting equal opportunities.

Many gay, lesbian, and bisexual applicants are unsure whether their sexuality may affect their future career. Although some within the profession may hold unsympathetic views, they are a decreasing minority. Be reassured that gay, lesbian, and bisexual doctors are found at all grades, across all specialties. Although many are happy to be open with colleagues about their sexuality, others still prefer to keep their personal lives private.

The Human Rights Act, which came into effect in 2001, offers greater protection to people who are not treated equally and the General Medical Council states that all applicants who have the potential to meet the learning outcomes set by the GMC should be considered without prejudice. The law and the intentions of professional bodies are laudable, but tackling the issue of diversity with respect to age, disability, ethnic origin, gender, and sexual orientation is challenging. However, the medical student population is becoming increasingly diverse and it is much easier for mature students and students with dependents, disabilities, and ill health to study medicine than it has been previously. Nonetheless students with particular needs should consider their choice of medical school carefully and advice is contained in later sections of this book to help guide you.

Don't be surprised if you have any doubts about studying medicine. Many potential medics will also be flirting with the idea of pharmacy, law, veterinary science, and other courses. Speak to some doctors – your own GP might be a start – and, if you can, arrange some work experience at your local hospital. Entering medicine is not a decision to be taken lightly or for the wrong reasons, and first-hand experience in a medical environment is the best way of determining whether you are actually suited to a career as a doctor before entering medical school.

Finally, the choice to study medicine should be your own. It will be you who needs to find the force of character to spend endless nights before exams revising. It will be you who needs to find the capacity to carry on studying for up to three years after the rest of your school friends have graduated and begun earning. Ultimately, the choices you make now will determine the rest of your working life. If you feel others are making these choices for you, now is the time to muster the courage and face up to those who put pressure on you.

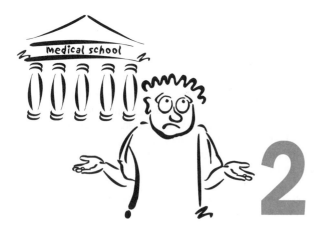

2

Life as a medical student

"Medical education is not completed at the medical school, it is only begun."

William H Welch (1850–1934)

"How unfair! Only one health, and so many diseases."

Victor Schlichter, attributed by his son Dr Andres J Schlichter,
Children's Hospital, Buenos Aires, Argentina

How am I going to be taught?

In the past, there was a view that medical students spent their first couple of years cramming a vast amount of knowledge without ever seeing a patient, and then emerged brainwashed, unable to think and unable to communicate. If this ever was the case, it is now certainly a thing of the past. Recommendations in the General Medical Council (GMC) report called *Tomorrow's Doctors* encouraged medical schools to reduce the emphasis on learning factual information and concentrate much more on developing the skills and attitudes needed to become a doctor. The foundations of factual knowledge established at medical school would then be built on whilst practising as a doctor. The report also recommended the introduction of special study modules (SSMs) to give students the chance to undertake projects of their own choosing. Alongside this, the GMC encouraged schools to adopt a more "problem-based" learning approach to teaching, where facts are taught within a framework of real-life clinical scenarios.

Developing research skills and encouraging intellectual curiosity and enthusiasm for learning, are now as important as knowledge. The emphasis is placed very firmly on producing graduates who will be life-long learners. The majority of medical schools have already changed their curricula so that older courses (in which science and clinical practice were taught separately) have given way to more "integrated" curricula. In other words, instead of learning subjects separately – for example anatomy, biochemistry, and physiology ("subject-based teaching") – students are more likely to learn about respiration, reproduction, diet, and metabolism in a more "system-based" approach.

Mikey's view: A day in the life of a preclinical student

Just another Tuesday. My alarm clock indicates that I have precisely 13 minutes to make the bed-to-medschool journey. Suffering from the throws of a fantastic hangover (courtesy of the Medics' Cocktail Party), I head with the feeling of impending doom towards the dissection room. Dissection with a hangover is not to be recommended, so a rigorous programme of sobering up is firstly employed! We start by reviewing the very systems we were abusing the night before – the liver and the GI system – followed by this week's objective: "Identify and display the key aspects of the female reproductive system." Sadly this will be rather tricky, considering our cadaver's history of a radical hysterectomy. I feel distinctly queasy; 90 minutes later we head to the legendary coffee bar with an unusual craving for a bacon sandwich.

Feeling nourished after satisfying those post-dissection munchies we arrive at the lecture theatre for 3 solid hours of lectures. The prospect is a remarkably unappetising combo of genetics and double reproduction. Having come in late I'm forced to sit at the front, clutching a bottle of water in one hand, fistful of paper in the other. With a disapproving raised eyebrow the lecturer starts. "Xeroderma pigmentosum"; sounds like a horrific cross between a photocopier and assorted farmyard animals!

The only thing that seems to be keeping me awake is the excitement that our Professor in physiology might beat his own personal best for the number of times he says "schematic" in a 50 minute lecture! Shortly after the peak of my excitement I feel a nudge in the shoulder. I knew I wasn't going to make it all the way through without falling asleep, but at least I don't snore! It's 2 hours in and I think I'm about ready to be turned. One can't be too careful, as pressure sores are a very real occupational hazard!

Lunch has to take a back burner today (now very thankful for that bacon sandwich), as next up is a communication skills assessment. This involves me taking a history from one of my female friends who is pretending to be a 76-year-old man with erectile dysfunction! How am I supposed to keep a straight face when it's all being recorded on video camera?

Still another 2 hours to go, but one of them is with my favourite lecturer in the skills lab. You'd be surprised how much fun you can have learning about urine! We're learning the basics of urinalysis, and how the presence of certain molecules in the urine indicates certain diseases.

(Continued)

(Continued)

The last session of the day is a physiology and pharmacology workshop. I took great delight in giving my housemate eyedrops which dilated one pupil and constricted the other, the net result being him falling off his chair. He took counsel in the fact that I was the subject for the next experiment, rumoured to be associated with gastrointestinal motility (ie movement)!

Heading home seems to fill everyone with energy, and the previously narcolepsy-prone students start planning the night ahead. I, however, will be sensible and stay in, as I have a hospital visit tomorrow and must be in for 8.30 am. Hospital visits are a real highlight, and one of the few opportunities us preclinical students get to play doctors and nurses. I get home, dust down the stethoscope and start rereading my notes. After some revision I feel I've definitely earned some time to myself. Rugby being my game, I head down to the pitch for a rather intense training session. Our team's doing really well this year, and there's an important tournament on the horizon. It's late when I get back, so a big group of us order takeaway and stay up for hours talking shop.

My alarm goes. It's 7.30 am, I'm running late and I appear to have slept in a pizza box. Damn my lack of will power! This hospital visit is going to be a real struggle...

In most schools, students will have some regular contact with clinicians and patients from the outset. The early years still have less clinical content and more lecture and laboratory teaching, but the traditional preclinical/clinical divide is dying. An important effect of these changes is that students need to be much more responsible for their own studies, and self-motivation and self-discipline is essential. Clinical skills laboratories have been introduced in most schools so that students can practise procedures and take exams on dummies and this helps to build confidence before going on the wards and carrying out the same examinations on patients. The balance between lectures, problem-based learning, SSMs, and clinical exposure will vary between schools and is worth considering carefully in order to help you choose the medical school which best suits your preferred style of learning.

Clinical work takes place in local teaching hospitals and district general hospitals (DGHs), which can be many miles away from the medical school. These "attachments" take you out of town, but getting away from the big city hospitals often provides the opportunity to be more involved in a team, gain more hands-on experience, and to ultimately learn more. Most schools provide free accommodation within the hospitals if commuting is not practical. Some schools will even allow overseas attachments in addition to the elective.

But I'm squeamish!

As you would imagine, there is a fair amount of blood and gore in medicine at various stages (for example physiology practicals, post mortems, dissection, and taking blood). Many students become used to this remarkably quickly. For others, it may take longer. It may surprise you to know that some doctors are still squeamish after many years of practice. If you are very concerned about how you might react, try to arrange some appropriate work experience at your local hospital.

I've heard it's really hard work!

Now that the emphasis is placed more on learning appropriate skills and attitudes, rather than cramming vast amounts of facts, the ability to be able to list off reams of detailed biochemistry or pathology is less important. Nonetheless there are still exams and the amount that a medical student is expected to know on graduation is still considerable. More importantly, the amount that you learn during your time at medical school will have a direct impact on your ability to perform as a young doctor, and the thought that the wellbeing of patients will shortly be in your hands, is an incredible motivation to work hard.

Medicine remains a very demanding course and friends studying for other degrees may have as many hours timetabled per week as you will have in one day. Attendance at lectures and practicals can last from 9 am until 5 pm every day, and regular evening and weekend study is essential. During the clinical years the hours spent in hospital are frequently much longer, and additional time is still needed for personal study and revision. There is no doubt that, if you want an easy option at university, medicine is not the right subject for you.

Mikey's view: A day in the life of a clinical student

The day starts with the rather unwelcome sound of the alarm clock at 6.30 am. It's still pitch black outside. After showering, dressing, making my lunch, and managing only half of my measly slice of toast, I'm already running late. I jump into the car at 8.10 am only to end up in a traffic jam! Typical!

After the 20 mile journey which has taken 45 minutes, I manage to make it to the outpatients' department where the urology clinic starts at 9 am. Actually, I'm "on take" today which means that I need to help receive the emergency patients into hospital. However, normally nothing really happens until after lunch when the GPs have had a chance to send some patients in. So, since I'm at the clinic before the surgeon and the junior doctors, I start to clerk all the new patients. Interestingly one has a hydrocele (a collection of fluid in the scrotum), which is a condition I have never seen before. At 11.30 am I have to leave, as radiology teaching is about to start.

Together with my fellow students, we await the arrival of the consultant; 20 minutes after the session was due to begin, a message is sent to say that our teaching has been cancelled as the consultant is too busy with an ultrasound list to teach us this morning. It is a nuisance as the clinic I had been at was really interesting.

It's midday and at the surgical admission unit things are quiet except for one patient who needs a cannula inserted (a cannula is a needle through which medication and fluid can be given). As I'm the only person who has turned up to the unit in the last 4 hours, the nurses jump on me as though I'm their oasis of hope and ask me to do it. My blood pressure's rising as I've been put on the spot and can't really say no – but it's a good chance to practise my clinical skills. I have to look in three different places for a vein, that I can use, as there doesn't seem to be a

(Continued)

9

(Continued)

decent one (they're not the greatest I've ever seen). However, I finally decide on the best. Confidence is definitely not oozing from me and I'm half expecting the vein to disappear but despite shaking, I manage to get it in.

The on-call registrar arrives on the ward, so I let him know the cannula is in and find out that there is an emergency appendicectomy about to take place. As a result I rush to eat my sandwiches whilst walking to theatres; it's 2.15 pm and I'm hungry. Once I've changed into scrubs, the surgeon asks me to "scrub up" and assist. He lets me hold things out of the way and cut a few stitches, and he talks me through the anatomy.

After completing the operation in 5 hours (it was complicated), a vascular surgeon informs me that there is a patient who is coming in with an abdominal aortic aneurysm, which is suspected to be leaking. An aortic aneurysm is when the main artery in the body is dangerously dilated (enlarged). As he is currently on the CT scanner showing images to identify any problems, I head towards the radiology department again. However, there is a hoard of people running in that direction too and when I arrive I find that the patient has had a cardiac arrest. As medical students, we're advised to observe such situations if we can before we qualify, however, I feel awkward standing in the corner watching the patient being resuscitated. A nurse spots me and asks me to count how long they've been resuscitating for. Although for once I'm being useful, the mêlée in front of me is a distraction. I don't want to be seen as a gawking "spectator". This isn't *ER* or *Casualty* – this is a real person dying in front of me. After 20 minutes, the patient is pronounced dead. People gradually exit one by one and I'm left not quite knowing what to do. Eventually I say a prayer for the patient and wonder if I'll still be doing the same thing when I've been to many more crash calls as a Junior House Officer.

The Senior House Officer comes over and asks me, "Is that the first person you've seen die?" "Yes," I say still trying to take the situation in. "If you need to talk about what you've just witnessed, then I'm happy to listen." "Thanks, but I'll be OK." At 9.00 pm (time flies), I make the decision to leave for home, recounting the events of the day. I'm exhausted and feel quite drained. After walking what seems like 20 miles through the hospital back to the car, driving home in the dark is not fun – I've barely seen the light today!

It's been a very busy day and I've been running on only some toast and a sandwich. Time for food! But before bed, preparation of some material must be done for a presentation tomorrow to one of the consultants. Sleep finally calls to me, at midnight, but I must be up early again for the post-take ward round…

In recent years, many medical schools have placed a greater emphasis on continuous assessment and a number have rearranged final exams so that they are taken over a longer period rather than all at once. Many students have found this to be a sensible development that has reduced a lot of the episodic pressure. Some, however, argue that this has only spread the pressure throughout the year; the increased number of exams can lead to exam fatigue and, at schools with more traditional courses, "finals" are still dreaded.

Is it fun?

Despite all these pressures, medical students have no trouble being sporty and sociable. In fact, we often excel at both. There is a wide mixture of students at every medical school and every group will contain a range of public school and state school, working class and middle class, medical family and non-medical family type backgrounds. You will be able to pursue your non-course interests as well as your studies. "Work hard and play hard" is the maxim that unites medical students, and the medical profession has an enviable community spirit – a "we're all in it together" attitude. Year groups vary in size but are often large (200+). Nonetheless, because everyone is doing the same course, you get to know your colleagues very quickly and very well. The downside of this is that medical students sometimes have a reputation for not mixing with students on other courses. It is also why we have the enviable reputation for the best social life! The common shared purpose amongst those studying medicine results in a closeness, which is one of the best aspects of life as a medical student.

Getting the balance right...

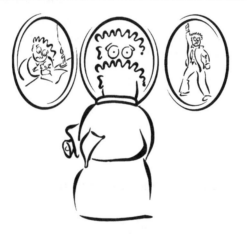

Maintaining a healthy balance between academic and extracurricular activities while at medical school is very important. One of the greatest benefits of university life is enabling students to develop as people as well as train to become doctors. A healthy interest in sport, music, theatre, or even just spending time relaxing with friends, will be important to your development as a well-balanced person, in addition to influencing your success as a doctor. Medicine is a demanding course and learning how to manage a healthy work-to-life balance early on will enable you to maintain it through the pressures of life as a doctor and increase your ability to cope with stress.

If you find that you have no time at all for socialising or pursuing a hobby, then something is wrong. Either you are working too hard and need to relax, possibly with the help of a stress counsellor, or you are living and/or studying in an inefficient way and would benefit from some coaching on organisation and study techniques. This is available at most universities in addition to a range of written resources including *How to Study* produced by the BMA. The importance of developing a well-balanced life during medical school cannot be overemphasised. Doctors are particularly vulnerable to stress-related conditions – depression, divorce, and alcohol abuse – and developing good practices as a student will help safeguard your health and happiness in the future.

It is also important to note that with the seemingly endless range of opportunities available at university and the active social life, it is easy to become involved in too much and find yourself pulled in too many directions. This situation can prove equally stressful and may cause academic difficulties. Most medical schools provide formative exams during the early terms, which should help you to gauge your academic progress. Use these as the excellent tool that they are to check that you have an appropriate balance between study and play, and adjust your activities as necessary.

Finally, it is worth bearing in mind that, at the end of your time at medical school, you will be applying for House Officer positions alongside a great number of other medical students with almost identical qualifications. Whilst there are enough jobs for everyone, if you have your heart set on a particular job it is helpful to have something that makes your curriculum vitae stand out from the crowd.

Can I combine medicine with pursuing another degree subject?

You can interrupt most courses to study for an extra "intercalated" degree, which is normally a medical science degree (BSc, BMedSci) undertaken during an extra year (or two) of study. This is particularly worthwhile if you are considering a career in research or academic medicine. Intercalated degrees are commonly taken after the second or third year, and entry policies vary between schools. They are compulsory in some, actively encouraged in others, and some allow students to intercalate by invitation only. In some schools where it is voluntary, as many as 50% of each year group intercalate at some stage in their studies. The main consideration to extending an already long course to complete an intercalated degree is the issue of financing an extra 12 months. At some schools tuition fees for the intercalated degree year are paid for, but you will still need to finance your living costs for an extra year.

Is it possible to travel abroad for any part of the course?

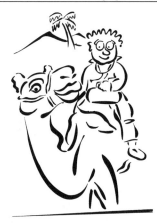

When people say that the world is your oyster, there is really no other profession that this applies to more aptly. Medicine truly is your passport to the world and doctors are trusted and welcomed in every corner, culture, and society. Medical schools have embraced this fact for many years now, and have incorporated a period within the medical curriculum dedicated to the students' own self-directed learning, termed an **elective**. The elective is usually over a period of between 8 and 12 weeks depending on which medical school you attend. To many students this means the chance to study overseas for a prolonged period. The elective is viewed as one of the major highlights of the undergraduate curriculum. Not only is it a fantastic learning experience but it is also a chance to escape the NHS and see parts of the world you have never seen before. Medicine is practised in diverse environments and settings, many of which are very different to the healthcare system that students will eventually enter. The elective allows the opportunity to experience how different healthcare systems contrast to our own. This may be the ultrasophisticated and technologically advanced system that exists in the USA or the humble resource-stricken system that exists in much of the developing world. Many students choose to place themselves in the latter environment because they are likely to gain a level of hands-on experience unavailable in more developed and regulated health services.

The timing of the elective varies between medical schools, but usually takes place during the clinical years so that students have a broad base of clinical knowledge before embarking on the elective period to maximise learning. All schools encourage the elective period to be used primarily as an invaluable learning resource and not just a holiday, although a holiday certainly can be incorporated. A number of schools require either clinical or academic research to be undertaken as part of the elective. Students decide to go on a particular elective depending on their interests and what they intend to achieve. For example, the adventurous may choose trauma in Johannesburg, whilst a student keen for a more relaxed experience may prefer to spend their elective in the Seychelles. With enough time and motivation, the opportunities are endless. For example, previous students have benefited from electives with NASA in the USA, the flying doctors in Australia, and the mountain rescuers in Nepal.

You do not have to go abroad for your elective and many students choose instead to organise an equally rewarding experience in the UK: perhaps delving into medical politics, carrying out a project at an academic or pharmaceutical research centre, or working with the team doctor at a football club. The elective really is what you make it. Generally, students organise their own elective with the assistance of the medical school, reports from previous students, and relevant elective literature. There really is no limit to what you can get out of your elective if you are prepared to put the effort in to organising it.

It can be expensive, depending on what you choose to do; however, there are numerous grants and prizes available which allocate money especially to help fund medical student electives, so, if you are well organised, it is often possible to obtain considerable financial support. Generally it is easier to obtain sponsorship and grants if your elective incorporates research.

Whatever you choose to do as part of your elective, the memories and experience that you will gain will be something you will never forget throughout your future career as a doctor.

In addition to electives, a few medical schools allow students to take one or more special study modules (shorter periods designed to allow students to study an area of particular interest) abroad. Furthermore a small number of universities allow medical students to take part in exchange programmes with other European nations for part of the course, and even to study a foreign language. This is called Erasmus and the ability to undertake these at each medical school is outlined in the second half of the book. If these opportunities interest you, then it is important to read the information for each medical school carefully as practices vary considerably and medical schools facilitating such opportunities are currently in the minority.

Is it wise to study medicine with a chronic illness or disability?

Medical school is tough. It is tough for everyone – even those who are 100% healthy. It places pressures on students academically, financially and emotionally. The decision to study medicine should not be taken lightly or without prior knowledge of those facts, particularly if you are chronically unwell or have a disability to contend with in addition to studying, and even more so if your health status fluctuates. This all sounds very daunting and may make you wonder whether you should even consider doing medicine. Believe it or not, you are probably the best-equipped individuals to tackle this vocational subject. The challenges and obstacles that you have faced are similar to experiences of those patients whom you will eventually serve. Your deeper understanding of illness is something that, although unfortunate, is invaluable to you and the profession. You really do know what it is like at both ends of the bed!

Medical schools are endeavouring to widen access to all potential students whatever their circumstances, and all medical schools are obliged to provide some form of pastoral care and support. However, the approach of the different medical schools to students with health problems and disabilities varies, as does the quality of the pastoral support available. Unfortunately, the "caring profession" isn't always as caring to its own. It is well worth considering these factors carefully when choosing which medical schools to apply to. This is explained in more detail in Chapter 3.

The Disability Discrimination Act 1995 requires that universities and medical schools take into account the needs of disabled students. They must provide statements about the facilities available for such students, which should include details such as access, the specialist equipment and counselling available, admission arrangements, and complaints and appeals procedures for disabled students. The Act applies in Northern Ireland with exceptions.

Because of the many demanding aspects to medical work, any disability that might impede clinical capability needs to be considered carefully. Depending on the disability or health problem, medical schools may require the applicant to have a skills assessment to ensure that they are fit to perform the tasks involved in becoming a doctor. This will focus on what the student can do, rather than what they can't do. Medical school faculties and occupational health services may be able to offer skills assessment and Deans of medical schools should be able to offer further information and advice. Students may be eligible for financial help, such as the disabled students' allowance. Following a publication by its Disabled Doctors Working Party titled *Meeting the Needs of Doctors with Disabilities*, the BMA launched a service for disabled medical students and doctors. This aims to provide information about aids, facilities, equipment, and financial help. It also puts disabled medical students and doctors in touch with each other. Further information may be obtained from the Medical Education Department of the BMA (see Further information section at the end of this book).

Despite the efforts of good medical faculties and the best intentions of the majority of students within a year, it is very easy to feel isolated when you are struggling with health problems. In order to reduce the impact of this on both your studies and your health, it is helpful to:

- accept your limitations – the most important rule;
- keep relevant people informed at all times, particularly when you feel that there may be a problem around the corner (medical faculties are able to help and to take circumstances into consideration if they know in advance);
- not to be afraid to ask for help – you are only human;
- always remember that your health is the most important thing – you don't want to end up next to the patients you are treating!

Medicine should be for everyone so do not be put off. The old mentality of "if it's too hot, get out of the kitchen" is gradually fading. As more people with illnesses and disabilities enter the profession, this attitude should disappear completely.

What about studying modioino as a mature student?

Over recent years there has been a dramatic increase in the number of applications from both graduate and mature students wanting to study medicine. Much of this has resulted from the introduction of 4-year fast track medical degrees for students who meet certain criteria, but even mature and graduate applications for traditional 5- and 6-year courses have increased. Previous experience and maturity are becoming increasingly valued and medical schools often view mature students as reliable and likely to "stay the course". These applicants have often achieved another degree or worked in professions allied to medicine, such as nursing, and many argue that these students have spent more time assessing whether they really want to be a doctor before taking the plunge into medicine.

In some undergraduate medical courses, as many as 15% of students are mature students, and the staff are used to dealing with their different needs. However, in other schools older students are a rarity. Indeed, until recently there were a significant number of medical schools that would not even accept applications from those aged over 40, 30, or even 25. Despite current initiatives against ageism, some medical schools continue to overtly dissuade applications from those who do not fit rigid age categories. The BMA continues to oppose age limits in UK medical education, and the success of both mature and graduate students means that more and more schools are welcoming applications from mature students.

Depending on their academic background, mature students may be eligible to join one of the fast-track graduate courses, whereas others may have to complete a **premedical** year. In these cases it is essential that applicants contact the admissions department of the medical schools to find out if there are specific entrance requirements. Graduate entry programmes (GEP) and premedical courses are discussed in more detail in Chapter 4.

A large proportion of mature students will be self-funding if they have previously completed undergraduate degrees, and consequently are likely to incur higher levels of debt than their younger colleagues. However, finances should not put you off applying to medical school if you are motivated and have a true desire to study medicine and become a doctor.

Before applying, it is worth listing honestly the pros and cons of returning to or continuing education for at least another 4 years. This is not a useless exercise as you can be sure that those interviewing you will want to be very sure of your motives and future plans. The BMA's graduate and mature students' group has identified specific issues that cause additional concern for those who are planning to change their lifestyle to study medicine. As a mature applicant you will need to consider:

- *Finance.* Can you afford it? What about your fees?
- *Partners and family matters*. What will this mean for them and for your relationship(s)?
- *Children, child care, and future pregnancies*. How will you fit them in?
- *Lifestyle changes* (such as loss of regular income, working unsociable hours). How will you cope if you are expected to live in a shared student flat?
- *Work/study mix*. Because of the demands of the course, most students are not able to work enough part-time hours to fund their courses.
- *Attitudinal challenges* (both your own and from teachers and fellow students).

When you are considering applying to medicine as a mature or graduate student, it is important to realise that attitudes towards mature students and the support systems in place to help with their needs, vary across UK medical schools. The majority of mature students thoroughly enjoy their time at medical school, but you must take responsibility for maximising your chances of satisfaction by choosing carefully the medical schools that you apply to.

Do many students manage to study medicine and care for dependents?

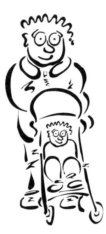

As if studying for one of the longest degrees, arguably involving some of the most mind-numbing memory work, was not enough, some students like to liven things up a bit by choosing to start their studies with a ready-made family of their own in tow. Others add the challenge of a pregnancy or two, to the otherwise all-too-quiet times we have as medical students.

In fact medical students have always done this. It's just that with more mature students these days, and greater choices for women in the workplace, it has become talked about, and rightly so. Scan the website of any of the university medical schools in the UK for their maternity policy for students and you'll be hard-pressed to find one. The sad fact is that when you approach your tutor to say that:

- you need to take time off because your child has chicken pox;
- your child care has fallen through and you'll be late for lectures;
- you want 6 months off because you're pregnant,

you are not likely to get the sort of treatment that you would get if you were at work. For example, we are aware of a case of a student whose daughter died but whose university tried to give her a fail mark for missing the OSCE she should have sat rather than being at her daughter's bedside in the paediatric intensive care. Another university offered such scant support to one pregnant student that she felt forced to leave and transfer to another medical school.

Nevertheless there are success stories. An increasing number of students manage to give birth and pick up on their studies by timing matters rather well to fit in with holiday periods (especially in the preclinical years when the holidays are longer). Others take a full year out and slot back into the next year. Indeed some think having a baby while a student is the best way to do it. After all it's not going to be any easier when you are a stressed out junior doctor, or when you're 15 years older and a consultant.

As more and more students with children or other dependents enter medicine, the provision of support and understanding will improve in the same way that flexible working patterns for doctors have had to radically improve as a result of the large number of both male and female practitioners who have demanded a better work-to-life balance. In the meantime enjoy your family *and* your time as a student. Remember many people are already doing just that – and the more students who do it, the more we can one day look forward to persuading universities to offer flexible degrees in the same way as there are flexible working arrangements.

Studying as an international student?

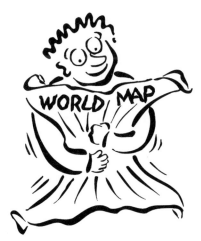

Medical students come from all over the world to study in the UK, with the majority coming from former Commonwealth nations in East Asia, South Asia, the Middle-East, and Africa. Students come from a wide variety of backgrounds and experiences, and find it a great opportunity to meet people and learn about cultures, which they would never have been able to in their own country.

Coming to the UK can be an overwhelming experience, as things can be quite unlike what you are accustomed to at home. From the type of food and entertainment, to the cultural values and way of life, you may find it very different from what you are used to. This can be a good thing. Britain is a very multicultural society, and it is generally easy to fit in and feel comfortable with your surroundings. It also means that you are likely to find at least one restaurant that serves a dish from your country, as there is more to British food than fish and chips!

It is generally a good idea to live on campus for the first year, so that you can get to know other students at your university and make new friends. It also gives you time to adapt to the British culture and way of life, before you move out into the "real world". Some universities allow international students to live on campus for up to 2 years. When students do move out, they tend to share accommodation with friends and colleagues whom they have met during their first year, which is the norm in the UK.

If you can get over the weather and the funny accents, the UK is an excellent place to undertake your undergraduate training. Most people involved in your training are keen to teach, the nurses and staff are helpful, and the patients are very friendly and willing for medical students to practise their clinical skills on them; all in the name of learning.

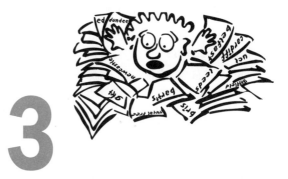

3

Applying to medical school

"Medicine, the only profession that labours incessantly to destroy the reason for its existence."

Sir James Bryce (1838–1922)

Choosing the right medical schools

Entrance requirements

Most medical schools require students to get A or B grades (mainly As) in at least three full A-level subjects (discounting general studies) or five Scottish Highers. Many schools also require the Scottish Certificate of Sixth Year Studies from applicants educated in Scotland. The entry requirements have gone up, and have remained high despite a downward trend in applicants (which has recently reversed). The average requirement is now AAB (AAABB). Chemistry is usually a compulsory requirement because the principles of chemistry are the key to understanding medical biochemistry, and it would be difficult to teach to the required standard during the course otherwise. Surprisingly, many schools don't insist on biology, although many medics have it as one of their A-levels. In most schools medical teaching covers elementary biology, and there may be supplementary classes for non-biologists during the first year.

Traditionally, the other subjects studied at A-level are sciences or mathematics, but many medical schools now acknowledge that students who pursue other subjects at school are not disadvantaged when they begin studying medicine. Some schools accept applications from students taking chemistry, another science subject and an arts A-level. However it is essential to check with each school before you make your final choices: don't rely upon what others have chosen before if your choices are a non-typical combination. Where possible, the key facts box reflects each medical school's requirements.

19

Health status

In addition to academic qualifications, you will also have to fulfil certain health-related entry requirements. Individual schools have different requirements, about which they will inform you if your application is successful, but in general you will need immunity against rubella and tuberculosis if you don't already have it. A majority of schools also require you to prove your hepatitis B status before admission.

Open days and further information

It is very important that you find out as much as possible about the medical schools to which you are considering applying. In Part 2 of this book we give you admission information and views and opinions for you to consider. Only by visiting the school and reading the prospectus and any alternative guides will you be able to assess the atmosphere and whether you will enjoy studying there. Remember, no one knows what life at medical school is like better than those already there. Don't be afraid to approach current medical students: we are generally a friendly bunch and would be more than happy to chat over a coffee about any aspect of medical school life.

Open days will help you decide whether you would prefer a medical school that is part of a larger university, on a campus or spread across a town, in a big city or near the countryside, and where you'd like to live should you accept a place there. It will also allow you to talk to the medics who are already there. Starting university can be a daunting experience, but if you know what to expect then you will be much more at ease. If you can't afford the cost of travelling, get a group together and ask if your school or college will sponsor a minibus or take a coach to an open day. Most open days take place in the summer after students have had their exams and before applications are due. It is better to go early, before students go on vacation, although there are clinical students milling around all year. Well-organised open days have a welcoming team to escort visitors from the station, and organise events, talks, tours, displays, and demonstrations. However, organisation varies greatly from school to school.

Some medical schools run intensive open days during which you may sample lectures. There are courses run commercially, giving application advice as well as an insight into life as a medical student. These can be expensive but may be a good way of helping you decide whether medicine is the right choice for you. Your careers tutor might be able to help you find out about these courses and open days.

If you can't attend an open day, there are a number of people you could write to. The Students Union can deal with enquiries and may have promotional material to send you. The Medical Faculty office should also be able to supply you with the name of the president of the Medical Society, the student group responsible for representing medics and organising sports and social events, so you can contact the students directly. BMA student representatives are always happy to answer questions, and they may be contacted through the medical school or via the BMA Medical Students Committee (see Further Information section).

Applicants with disabilities

As medicine is a vocational course, medical schools do not tend to accept students unless they are confident that the applicant has the potential to meet the requirements of the preregistration house officer year. This year is based on a series of learning outcomes, details of which can be obtained from the General Medical Council. Where an applicant has a disability or chronic health problem, which may impact on their study, good admission practice suggests that medical schools should first assess an applicant without reference to their illness or disability. If the school is happy to offer that student a place but feels that clarification of the health challenge is necessary, the applicant should undergo an occupational health assessment to determine whether they would be physically and mentally capable of meeting the learning outcomes of the preregistration year.

Although the attitude of most medical schools is changing, and some have in place very positive practices, it can still be difficult for a student with a significant disability to gain a place at medical school. When considering which medical schools to apply to, you should speak to the medical faculties prior to applying in order to gain an impression of their attitudes. The good medical schools will have past or present students with health problems or disabilities with whom they can put you in touch, and the medical faculty personnel will be encouraging and keen to help. It can also be very helpful to try and arrange a meeting with either the Dean or the Admissions Officer prior to applying.

There are a number of organisations which might also help – in particular, SKILL, the National Bureau for Students with Disabilities. For their address and details of support for people who feel that they are being treated unfairly look in the Further Information appendix of this book.

Mature applicants

Do your research! Much will be gained from making contact with the admissions tutors at those medical schools that you are interested in applying to. The attitude of the admissions staff and the tone of the welcome that you receive can provide clues as to the possible reactions to your application. Do not forget that, as a mature applicant, you are entitled to send "supporting material" to the admissions teams in addition to your UCAS form – do not just limit this to a CV. Discuss with the school the form that this should take. Determine what will make your case most effective. You can use letters of support, details of relevant courses, work experiences, etc. The newer medical schools have been reported to be much more welcoming to those who have had a career elsewhere or who do not fit the typical school-leaver applicant's profile. Some older establishments, however, are also keen to recruit more mature students. Contact the schools directly. Read the prospectuses carefully.

Above all, be sure that this is what you want to do. At interview, be prepared to be grilled as to the reasons why you want to change your life at this point in time. Remember, nothing sounds as good or as convincing as the truth!

Applicants with dependents

Before selecting where to apply, talk to the universities on your short list. Find out:

- whether it has any medical students with dependents that you can talk to;
- its policy on maternity leave for students;
- whether child care is provided, and whether it is subsidised for students;
- whether there is specific support available for mature students or students with dependents;
- whether there are any special hardship grants for students with dependents.

Choose universities that are encouraging and positive towards you. The admissions tutor's response to your initial enquiries will speak volumes about that university's potential attitude towards you in the future. Remember, mature women students with young children are more likely than any other group to abandon their course and it doesn't take many brain cells to work out why.

International applicants

The first step for a prospective international student considering studying in Britain is to determine the cost of education in its entirety, (including tuition fees, equipment, books, and living expenses), as this can be very high. The next step is to find out if your country of origin offers any loans, scholarships, or grants to study abroad, as some governments do offer financial relief for their citizens to experience medical training in another country. It is also worth finding out if the university that you are considering offers any scholarships to international students. The best way to find this out is to contact the university directly and ask. British Embassies or High Commissions and your own country's education authorities may also be able to advise you on grants and scholarships.

After reading the university prospectus, you should contact the school and clarify and verify any information, as the situation can change, that may influence your decision to attend a particular school. The British Council will have information about UK universities and medical schools. It will also be able to guide you on whether your qualifications are recognised in the UK. If you are not studying UK-examined A-levels, then contact the admissions office at the medical school to check whether your subject choices and qualifications are acceptable. There are growing links between overseas medical schools and UK schools, and you may be able to do some of your studies in the UK even if you don't get a full-time place on the course. If you are applying to medical schools in other countries you might want to enquire about this.

Applicants from outside the UK must also apply via UCAS and should follow the instructions in the *UCAS Handbook*. You can get copies of the UCAS information from British Council offices or by writing to UCAS. Many schools and colleges will order supplies for you.

Gap years

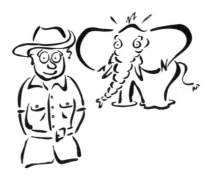

Many sixth-form students defer entry to university for 12 months. Gap years are looked on favourably by most colleges and universities. The majority, however, expect you to use the time profitably by working and/or travelling. It is important that you check the medical school's attitude before you apply if you intend to defer entry. Time out between school and university is not just for those who have the money for a "round-the-world" air ticket: a well-planned gap year will give you time to think about how to get through university and let you assess what you want to get out of the next five or more years. Time spent well will boost your confidence and broaden your experience. This can have a very positive effect on your performance. Student debt is increasing all the time. You could try to save some money and be in better financial shape for your eventual university career. A gap year may also be used to gain some more work experience in health care, although there is no need to overdo it.

Note: A minority of institutions don't approve of gap years. It is best to check the attitude of the individual college(s) to which you are thinking of applying.

The application process

The UCAS form

Medical schools only accept applications made through the Universities and Colleges Admissions Service (UCAS). Read through the *UCAS Handbook* and follow the advice closely. Make several drafts of your UCAS form before finalising your application. Your careers tutor at school or college will be able to help you fill in the form. If you do not have a careers tutor try and find someone else to read through a draft version for you before you write it up – perhaps a family friend or your work experience supervisor. When you do write it up, remember to make it accurate and legible.

The most important part of the form is the personal statement. This is your chance to stand out from the crowd and make the admissions tutors want to interview you. What you write will go a long way towards determining how many medical schools offer you an interview or a place. The comments below apply equally to electronic and paper applications.

You can expect – not surprisingly – that the medical school will want to know why you want to study medicine and, as there is so much competition, you must seize this opportunity to demonstrate your commitment to joining the profession. For example, you may want to try to describe what drives you to pursue a career in medicine. Medical schools will want to be sure that you know what you are getting yourself into, and so it is very important to demonstrate how you have gone about trying to understand what a medical career will entail. However, don't take too much space to do this, as it will be at the expense of other important information. The challenge is to do this effectively with supporting evidence of a well-balanced character – for example, a hospital portering job or regular visiting to a local old people's home, along with captaining the school netball team or editing the school magazine. These examples will prove to them that you are a good candidate and that you are well rounded in your interests.

It should be clear from the information supplied by your school or college whether you have the potential to get the grades, so the personal statement must show you as a potential asset to the medical school and, later, the medical profession. They will be looking for:

- signs of good interpersonal skills
- evidence of a social life

- details of your interests/hobbies
- any notable achievements.

You could mention:

- sports achievements
- academic prizes
- organisational or supervisory positions of responsibility
- voluntary work, part-time work
- musical or travel interests
- projects that you have particularly enjoyed or unusual hobbies.

If you are deferring entry for a year you should explain how you are going to use your time.

There is no need to explain your choice of A-levels/Highers unless you have something interesting to say about them, for example: "I am studying computing as an A-level as I think it may lie at the heart of medicine in the future." Don't be afraid of making bold comments as long as you can justify them. They also offer signposts for interviewers that can be prepared for before an interview (see The Interview section below).

If you are called for an interview, the panel will question you on the contents of this section, so don't lie or exaggerate your interests or achievements. Remember, you may be asked to talk about any of the things you mention, so be truthful – it will probably show very quickly if you have embellished too much!

Admissions staff read hundreds of UCAS forms, and if yours stands out then you will have a better chance of being called for interview. The admissions tutor will want to know that you are prepared for what a career in medicine entails, and that you have realistic expectations, so by the time you post your application form you should have done your research and thinking.

You can use this book to help you decide which schools to apply to, but don't put an overt preference in the application. Another medical school may dismiss your application if they think that you will turn down their offer, and, if you change your mind or your first choice medical school do not offer you a place, you will have limited your options. Also, think carefully about how your statement will appear to an admissions tutor reading it in his or her office. If you express a passionate interest in premiership football, an admissions tutor at Peninsula might think you would not enjoy being miles from any of the top clubs and not offer you an interview. Equally, an application to a Scottish medical school might appear eminently sensible from a student interested in ceilidh dancing.

When to apply

Apply as early as possible, but do not rush your application form. Importantly, remember to submit it well before the appropriate deadlines, bearing in mind that applications to certain universities may be earlier than others (such as Cambridge and Oxford). The UCAS guide and website give you all the details. You can submit your application electronically. You may receive replies from medical schools virtually as soon as you apply or you may be kept waiting until the last week that offers can be made. Either way do not read too much in to it. Some schools may make a conditional offer on your application alone, whereas others will conduct many rounds of interviews before they make offers or rejections. You may think that you have been forgotten – this is very unlikely, but it does happen. If you are in doubt, and the deadline is approaching, contact the admissions office. You can arrange for UCAS to acknowledge receipt of your form, and you will be given an application number so that you can check its progress if you feel it is taking too long. Admissions offices will be very busy during this time, but a telephone call may put your mind at ease even if they can't give you a decision on your application.

The interview

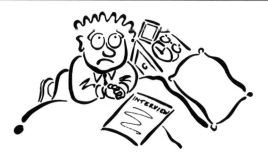

If you are called to an interview, make sure that you have done your homework thoroughly. The key to a good interview is excellent preparation and lots of practise. Prepare draft answers to the questions that you are likely to be asked. Do not learn these by heart, as you will sound rehearsed, but by thinking ideas through before the interview you will be prepared for possible pitfalls and will have thought about the most important information that you want to include. Practise interviews with anyone who is willing to spare 10 minutes. Ask them to suggest ways of improving your answers or style. This will help you to be more relaxed when it comes to the real thing.

Interviewers will be looking at your UCAS form for inspiration. They will probably be interested in what is special and unusual (but not weird) about you: they would be fascinated to find out what drove you to do a llama herding course in South America during your gap year – tell them! Reread your personal statement and anticipate the kinds of questions that you might be asked. This is where your personal statement and your interview should mesh. Place signposts in your personal statement that interviewers can pick up on and question you about. Remember, they may be interviewing 40 people in one day, and you can make it easier for them by doing this. You should also keep up to date with medical news stories and developments, as these may be the subject of some questioning.

Dress smartly and arrive in good time. If you are going to be shown around the medical school, remember that this is an opportunity to ask current students any questions that you might have. Don't feel obliged to ask any questions in the interview, and don't ask questions that are already answered in the prospectus. In some ways an interview is a chance for the medical school to assess the potential it has recognised in your application form. It is not an academic test. Treat it as an opportunity to show that you are serious about your career choice, and that you will be a future asset to the profession.

If you do not think that the interviewers are asking you the questions that will allow you to shine, it is possible to use an answer to one question to lead on to the subject that you would like to talk about. For example, if they have not asked you about your sporting activities, then you can reply to a question about why you have applied to their university to talk about the excellent sporting opportunities available and how that would suit you well in your endeavours as a County Junior Athlete. Whilst it is not a good idea to start rambling off on a complete tangent, a skilful interviewee can heavily influence the direction of the interview.

Most importantly, enjoy your interview. It is an opportunity for the panel to get a feel for the sort of person you are. Be polite and respectful, but be yourself. If you don't agree with something, then say so, as long as you can justify your disagreement logically and concisely. Although it is difficult to predict the exact questions that you will be asked, a number that reoccur time and time again include:

- Why do you want to be a doctor? Why a doctor and not a nurse?
- If you are so fascinated by the human body, why don't you do biology or physiology instead?
- Why do you want to come to this medical school?
- What can you offer the medical school?
- What are the most important characteristics of a doctor? What makes a good doctor?
- Do you know about the medical career structure?
- Do you know what sort of doctor you would like to be?
- What is the one thing you would like to change about the health service?
- Please give me three of your strengths and three of your weaknesses? (Be careful when selecting your weaknesses – you do not want to be so honest that it counts against you. An example would be "I'm prone to being too much of a perfectionist at times. I think that I will have to work on this during my time at medical school so that I can manage the demands of being a doctor without getting too frustrated at the lack of time to do everything quite as well as I would like").
- Please describe a situation when you worked in a team?
- Please describe a time when you have had to make a difficult decision? What is the hardest decision you've ever had to make?
- Questions that try to elicit whether you can think from a doctor's AND a patient's perspective.
- You may be given an ethical situation that you have to go through. (Here interviewers may be looking for characteristics such as teamwork, dealing with uncertainty.)
- You may be asked to talk about a life-changing event.

What if I don't get in?

The number of applicants to study medicine dropped by more than 3% in 2000 to 9291, but increased to 11 030 in 2002. In spite of this and the increased number of places, medical schools in the UK are still vastly oversubscribed. There are often 10 applicants for each place, and only a small fraction of them will make it to interview, selected on the basis of their UCAS forms and references; even fewer will get a place. Oxford and Cambridge have fewer applicants per place, which might mean that, although the academic requirements are high, you stand a slightly greater chance of at least being called to interview. However, not getting a place to read medicine is simply a reflection of the pressure on places and not a great indictment of your character and abilities. Even if you maximise your chances of being selected for interview, you may still be unsuccessful in your application.

You need to know what to do next. First, think long and hard! Do you still want to study medicine? Medical schools try to select people who will make good doctors and who have the right ability and motivations for studying medicine, but even so some students choose to leave mid-course and others fail exams. The interview panel has a responsibility to make the right decision for the medical school, and you have a responsibility to yourself and your potential future patients to make sure you are making the correct choice. Examine your reasons for wanting to study medicine. If in doubt, or if you have felt pushed in the direction of medicine, it might be better to look at different courses or careers.

If you still want to study medicine, then start by asking yourself why you weren't successful in your application. Did you get an interview? If you did, your school might be able to get some feedback from the medical school. This is unlikely to be in depth, but might give you some useful information. Discuss the prospect of your chances with teachers. Reflecting on your disappointment at this stage may prove difficult, but it is in your interests to be honest and realistic. Think about the possibility of following another course, whether in a related field – for example physiology, pharmacy, physiotherapy, biochemistry – or something totally unrelated. Most universities offer places on degree courses through "clearing". If your grades are good then many other courses will be open to you. It is possible to reapply to read medicine, but some schools will only consider a second application if you applied there first time round. If you do reapply, your A-level results should be at least as good as the estimates that your school originally made. There are some schools that will consider candidates who are resitting but others do not. Save your own time and energies by asking your preferred schools if they would accept an application from you. This could prevent you from wasting future UCAS choices. It is only advisable to resit exams if you are sure about getting A grades the second time around or if there were extenuating circumstances, such as bereavement or serious illness, in the months preceding your A-levels first time around.

There are a growing number of places available for graduates to read medicine, which means that you could do a degree and decide after graduation whether you still want to become a doctor. Some students start university studying a parallel course, such as physiology, and then apply to switch to medicine at the end of the first or second year when the university has had a chance to measure their potential and character. These students would still have to start medicine from the first year though, and this method of entry is very rare and should not be relied on. Graduates usually follow the full undergraduate medical course unless they can be exempted from part of it because of the nature of their first degree (for example, biochemistry or dentistry). Graduates with a purely arts background at A-level or degree could try to take a medical foundation year (premed year) before the medical course proper. This is not available at all institutions. Graduate entry, however, is one of the ways into a career as a doctor. The BMA, and many other interested parties, have recognised the desirability of graduate entry and, as more places are being reserved for graduates, it is sensible to consider this route as an option.

4

Graduate and premedical courses

"The work of the doctor will, in the future, be ever more that of an educator, and ever less that of a man who treats ailments."

Lord Horder

"If you want something done right, you have to do it yourself. This especially includes your health care."

Dr Andrew Saul

Not everyone knows from an early age that medicine is the career for them. Many students gain A-levels or even degrees before deciding to pursue a career in medicine. This section gives course information for these students, along with details of application procedures.

Graduate entry programmes (GEP)

Nowadays more and more entrants to medical school have already completed an undergraduate degree and may be eligible to undertake a 4-year fast-track graduate entry programme (GEP). In fact, many of the Government's planned new places are being reserved for graduates as schools develop graduate-only courses. Medical schools view graduates as reliable and likely to "stay the course". These mature students have done something else with their lives – often another degree – before taking the plunge into medicine and, it can be argued, have spent more time assessing whether they really want to be a doctor. In some schools as many as 15% of students are graduate entrants, and the staff are used to dealing with their different needs.

University	Places	Course details
Birmingham	40	• 4-year medical course open to graduates of life science subjects with minimum 2:1 in first degree; sound knowledge in chemistry • students are taught in a separate stream for the first 2 years, before joining the specialty clinical rotations of years 4 and 5 of the 5-year MBChB degree
Bristol	19	• 4-year medical course requiring at least a 2:1 BSc with biomedical science in first degree
Cambridge	20	• 4-year medical course open to graduates of **any** discipline • all candidates are required to take the Medical and Veterinary Admissions Test (MVAT), after application and before interview
GKT	40	• 4-year medical course open to graduates of **any** discipline with at least a 2:1 in their first degree • suitable candidates for the course take a written aptitude test; interviews offered on the basis of the application form and the aptitude test results
Leicester/ Warwick	164	• 4-year medical course open to graduates with at least a 2:1 degree in a biological science or degrees with the appropriate levels of biology
	64	• 4-year medical course open to graduates with at least a 2:1 degree in health sciences
Liverpool	40	• 4-year medical course open to graduates with at least a 2:1 in biomedical and health sciences and from approved social care professions • the programme covers the first 2 years of the 5-year course in one academic year (expanded by an extra 10 weeks)
Newcastle	95	• 4-year medical course open to graduates of **any** discipline • offers to graduates will be conditional on at least a 2:1 or a 2:2 degree combined with a PhD • applications from those whose prior professional experience matriculates them for entry are welcomed • candidates interviewed for the accelerated programme are likely to be required to sit an admissions test, the results of which will form part of the overall selection process
Nottingham/Derby	91	• 4-year medical course open to graduates of **any** discipline who have obtained or are predicted to obtain, a minimum of Bachelors (Honours) degree classified 2:2 or better • applicants have to complete the GAMSAT test (this tests knowledge, reasoning skills, and communication across a range of disciplines) • those who achieve the highest marks will then be offered a structured interview for a place on the course

(Continued)

(Continued)

University	Places	Course details
Oxford	30	• 4-year graduate entry course for biological science graduates • a special 2-year transition course is taught at the hospital site, with college-based tutorials, leading to the final 2 years of the standard clinical course • applicants must complete a Biomedical Admissions Test
Southampton	40	• 4-year medical course open to graduates of **any** discipline with at least a 2:1 in their first degree • there is no entrance examination or interview
St Bart's	40	• 4-year medical course open to graduates with at least a 2:1 degree in a science or health-related studies degree • those who meet the criteria are allocated a random number and a computer generates a random list of numbers • the first 140 sit the Personal Qualities Assessment (PQA) test • those who perform satisfactorily in the PQA will be invited to attend an interview – offers are made to those who score best at interview • priority for 14 places are given to applicants from the Biomedical Sciences, Materials Science and Engineering courses at Queen Mary, University of London
St George's	70	• 4-year medical course open to graduates in **any** discipline • they must have or be predicted at least a 2:2 degree in any discipline • applicants have to complete the GAMSAT test – those who perform well in the test are offered an interview
Swansea	30	• 4-year medical course open to graduates of **any** discipline with at least a 2:1 in their first degree • applicants have to complete the GAMSAT test – those who perform well in the test are offered an interview

The number of GEPs available has increased dramatically over the last few years. These courses vary in their entry requirements so it is worth investigating thoroughly. Most universities requirements include at least a 2.1 degree in a science-based or health-related subject. However, many also take students from any discipline. In addition, the majority of schools require applicants to undertake an entrance exam, the results of which are used to offer interviews. Details on the GEPs offered by universities can be seen in the table above. However, students are encouraged to contact the relevant universities for more information.

Most self-funding students and many graduate entrants will incur higher levels of debt than their younger colleagues. However, finances should not put you off applying to medical school if you have a true desire to become a doctor. Students on approved 4-year graduate entry courses are eligible for an NHS bursary from year 2 of studies onwards. Although many schools do not normally consider applicants over 30 years of age, some graduate programmes have no upper age limit. However, it must be noted that competition for places on these programmes is high, and the number of spaces available is relatively small.

Premedical courses

While most medical degrees last 5 or 6 years, some schools offer a premedical year. This year, which is intended as a foundation year in basic sciences, gives students with good non-science A-level grades (and some non-science graduates, if there is not an appropriate GEP) a way into the medicine degree course.

There are significant variations in the way these courses are taught and organised, and the exact nature of the premedical course varies from school to school. At some schools, students who complete the year successfully can apply to join the medical degree course, whereas at others there is automatic transfer to the first year of the 5-year course.

Premedical courses may be taught within the medical faculty or in other university departments. Exemptions from parts of the course may be offered if that subject has already been studied to a sufficient level, and some schools offer a choice of subjects studied. In addition, certain schools also specify that particular science subjects are needed at GCSE/Standard Grade level.

Medical schools offering premedical courses are listed below, along with some course details. However, students are encouraged to contact the relevant universities for more information.

University	Places	Course details
Belfast	5	• course for students with more broadly based qualifications than A-levels, eg Scottish Highers or Irish Leaving Certificate • students attend first-year courses in chemistry, physics and biological science
Bristol	10	• students who have not studied science at A-level are admitted into a 'preliminary year' where they can acquire the necessary science background before commencing the 5-year programme • the premedical year is spent studying the equivalent of A-levels in chemistry, biology and physics • premedical students study alongside predental students
Cardiff	12	• premedical course is restricted to applicants who cannot meet the programme requirements for direct entry to the 5-year programme • it is a modular programme and studies centre on the chemical and biological sciences, or other subjects selected according to the student's prior qualifications
Dundee	Up to 14	• course is designed to meet a demand and, if this demand is not apparent, it is not important if the number of students in the premedical year is very small • the year is provided for applicants with good passes in non-science subjects and is not available for applicants whose passes in science subjects do not meet requirements for first year.

(Continued)

(Continued)

University	Places	Course details
Edinburgh	No set number	• Dundee's premed students join with first-year BSc courses in chemistry, biology and physics • premedical year is an extra year of study for applicants who do not have the subject entrance requirements for the 5-year programme • it consists of selected courses from the first year of the Biological Sciences course • successful students continue on to the 5-year course
GKT	40	• premedical year is an extra year of study for applicants who do not have the subject entrance requirements for the 5-year programme, but achieve the academic requirements • applicants with qualifications not considered for the 5-year programme may also apply • course covers biology, chemistry, physics, and maths • students study alongside those taking BSc degrees
Manchester	18–20	• Premedical/Predental Programme occupies a single year and is designed for students who do not have the required science qualifications for direct entry into 5-year programme but have achieved good grades, in mainly arts subjects or, in the case of mature students, have a good arts degree • students learn fundamentals of biology, physics, and chemistry in an environment which has a relevance to clinical medicine – this is achieved with problem-based learning cases, theatre events, and skills sessions • entry to the next year of the medical course is automatic on satisfactory completion of this year
Newcastle	10–15	• premedical year is open only to applicants without a science background • students study a combination of chemistry, biological sciences, and medical data handling
Sheffield	15	• premedical science foundation course is a modified 'Access to Science' course tailored to give students with a non-scientific background the necessary basic scientific knowledge to undertake the medical course • course is designed to prepare students for the first part of the medical course, and is studied at Barnsley College • visits are made to the medical physics, clinical chemistry, and anaesthetic departments of a local hospital • students also gain basic scientific knowledge through studying biology, chemistry and physics

5

Funding your way through

"The physician should not treat the disease but the patient who is suffering from it."

Maimonides

What to expect

Money is an issue close to most students' hearts, and medical students are no exception. Government reforms of the higher education funding system, such as the introduction of tuition fees and the abolition of maintenance grants in 1998, have meant that the issue of debt is one that is affecting many more students than in previous years.

A recent BMA report (*Annual Survey of Medical Students' Finances 2002/2003*) found that the average total debt among final-year students was over £17 000. More than 3% of final-year medical students had debts in excess of £20 000. Although this may seem quite daunting, you shouldn't let it put you off studying medicine. Yes, you are likely to be in more debt after graduation than someone who takes a 3-year degree course, but this is balanced by excellent future career prospects and good job security. Medical student intake reflects all sectors of society. If you are not supported by wealthy or generous parents, **you won't be alone** in being in debt, and it won't be forever. There are currently more jobs than there are doctors in the UK, and this trend looks set to continue for some time, so unemployment after graduation is not really an issue. Most medical graduates pay off their debt within 5 years of graduation, which helps to explain why bank managers tend to be very welcoming to medics!

Medicine, depending on where you choose to study it, can take you between 4 and 6 years, so you will have to consider how you will support yourself for that time. The first 2 years are often the least financially demanding, as a great proportion of your year will be holidays. For many, this allows living at home for half the year and saving some costs; also, you will have plenty of time to earn cash in the holidays, if you want or need to. It gets a little trickier in your clinical years (when you spend more time in hospital): a total annual holiday of 6 weeks is considered good! During this time you'll have to pay for rent and food for the whole year, and it becomes difficult to find paid work when you have only 6 weeks off. Some students get part-time jobs during term time, although it is not always easy to fit this in. There are many kinds of expenses involved in studying medicine, and debt is likely to stare you in the face earlier than you might anticipate. Medicine is different from almost any degree course and there are several additional expenses: for example, there will be many expensive books to buy – you could spend at least £150 per year – and medical equipment, such as stethoscopes, can cost around £60. You will also need some smart clothing once you're in hospitals regularly. This is to make you look and feel like part of the medical profession, and to help you gain the trust of your patients.

The financial issue of the moment is the proposed introduction of "**top-up fees**", which could mean that tuition fees could be as much as £3000 per year. Student bodies and the BMA are opposed to their introduction, as they will discourage people from attending university because they simply cannot afford it. The BMA's Medical Students Committee (MSC) is campaigning vehemently to prevent their institution and to relay this to central Government. The Government's recent White Paper on Higher Education outlines proposals for funding higher education in the future. More information is available on the BMA website but changes are not likely to come into force until 2006. Please contact individual universities to find out the exact situation – even though they may have no plans to charge additional fees at present, will they expect you to pay if they are introduced halfway through your course?

The obvious question is "How will I pay for all this?" The first port of call for many people will be parents, guardians, or family, who may be able to give you something towards the cost of studying. If they are generous, the problem is solved, but if not (which applies to most of us) then there are government loans, bank loans, overdrafts, and many other ways to fund yourself through university.

The type of funding that you receive depends on a couple of factors: where you live in the UK and whether you have a previous degree. Funding arrangements for Scottish and graduate students will be discussed later in the chapter.

The year 2002 saw the introduction of the NHS bursary, which means funding arrangements are different depending on which year of the course you are in, but this will be explained in the following sections.

Costs associated with studying medicine

Tuition fees

Since October 1998, students have been required to contribute towards the cost of their education. For 2003/2004 the maximum home students had to pay was £1125 per year. If your family income is below a certain level (approximately £20 500 pa), you will not be expected to pay tuition fees at all. The full amount will only be payable if your parents' residual income is in excess of £30 502. Tuition fees make up a proportion of the cost of your tuition, the rest is made up by your Local Education Authority (LEA) in the form of mandatory and discretionary awards.

The BMA's MSC persuaded the Government that special consideration needed to be given to medical students because of the length and expense of the course, and the Department of Health agreed to pay tuition fees for medical students from year 5 of study onwards. This also applies to students doing premedical or intercalated years. This means that you will only pay tuition fees for the first 4 years of your course.

Living costs

Money for accommodation, food, transport, books, and beer will come from parental contributions, maintenance loans, and, invariably banks. The amount of maintenance loan to which you will be entitled will depend on where you study and what year you are in. Loans are administered by the Student Loans Company: 25% of the loan is means tested and will depend largely upon your parents' income. The maximum loan available in 2003/2004 for students outside London was £4000 and for those in London £4930, with smaller amounts being available to students living at home. Student loan repayments will be paid in instalments after graduation, once your income is over £10 000 per year. For medics, repayments will begin during the first house officer job, which will generally be a few months after finals. There is extra money available for courses that last longer than 30 weeks. In response to campaigns by the MSC, the Department of Health has agreed to provide means-tested non-repayable bursaries for medical students from year 5 onwards, for which students will be able to apply in addition to student loans. Students taking premedical and/or intercalated years will also be able to apply for this from year 5 onwards.

Travelling expenses

Most of the teaching on medical courses takes place on clinical attachments in hospitals and GP surgeries. These can be quite a distance from your main medical school base, meaning that travelling expenses can be considerable. Some medical schools offer travel expenses reimbursement, but this is by no means universal; the best way to find out is to contact the medical schools to which you are thinking of applying. It is expected that most students will fund travel expenses out of maintenance loans, although some may be claimed back from your LEA. The rules currently state that you can claim back travelling expenses incurred in attending clinical placements, although the first £265 must be borne by you. The amount you receive will be means tested. You should contact your local LEA to find out the arrangements for claiming expenses, and keep receipts and a record of journeys made to help your claim.

Boosting your funds

High-street bank

In addition to the maintenance loan, a bank overdraft is likely to be required. Surviving at medical school makes this an almost essential part of your finances. Most banks and building societies offer students special terms on bank accounts. These normally include interest-free overdrafts. Keeping your bank manager happy by not exceeding the agreed overdraft limit is good practice, and also helps you avoid penalty charges and punishing interest rates. If you want to extend your overdraft, go and discuss it with the manager face to face. The bank wants your custom because you will have a good job at the end of your university career, and they are experienced at helping students out with money problems. Banks are more likely to be generous and sympathetic with students who keep them informed than those who constantly surprise them. If you need more cash than an overdraft gives you, then you may need a loan. Look around to make sure you have accessed all other sources of funding before you take out a loan, for example hardship funds and charitable funds (see below). Banks can be willing to accept begging letters and IOUs from medics, and many have specially tailored loans of up to £20 000 for medical students.

Remember, however, that the debt you incur will have to be paid back regardless. Do not be blasé – heaven forbid that through illness, failure, or other unpredictable acts you do not qualify and are unable to repay your debts. Such instances are rare, but it would be irresponsible for us to overlook these possibilities. Make sure you fully understand the terms of the loan and shop around for the best deal. Don't just go to the bank you have an account with – it won't necessarily offer you the best deal.

Charities

There are literally hundreds of educational trust funds and charities in the UK, many of which support medical students. They tend to be open to mature and graduate students rather than school leavers, but it may be worth trying to find some funding from these sources. General directories of charitable trusts are available in the reference section of most public libraries and some are listed in the Further Information section of this book. Spending time searching through the lists and applying for grants may be to your advantage. Many small trusts have bizarre criteria for offering awards, and you may be surprised to find that, by meeting the unusual requirements, you can get help towards your expenses.

Access funds, hardship funds, and hardship loans

Universities receive money from the Government to help students in the poorest financial shape. Applications for the money are processed locally and policies on how these funds are distributed vary widely from school to school. It is important to be aware that this money is available.

Work

For the majority of medical undergraduates, working during vacations in the early part of the course is a necessity. As well as casual work in bars and restaurants, many students work as healthcare assistants and medical secretaries. Work can usually be arranged through the teaching hospital or other local hospitals. The experience of working in a hospital environment in a role other than as a medical practitioner can be very valuable. As the course progresses, however, the holidays get shorter as term time extends and periods of elective study intervene, and it then becomes more difficult to find employment for these shorter periods. You might consider taking a part-time job during term. The medical course is undoubtedly challenging and demands a lot of your time in studying, no matter how gifted you are. Because of this, some medical schools discourage students from working during term. They cannot actually prevent you from doing so, but be warned that they may take a dim view. Check out the school's attitude with the medics on open days. Do not let a job get in the way of studies.

Some medical students sign up to one of the Armed Forces medical cadet schemes. A "salary" is paid to cadets for 2–3 years. In return for this support during undergraduate training, cadets serve as an officer with, for example, the Royal Army Medical Corps, for a minimum period of duty (normally 6 years after full qualification). The income cadets receive is very generous compared with other students' incomes, but the *quid pro quo* is the 6-year short service commission. You will continue to practise as a doctor, but the Ministry of Defence will require you to support military initiatives anywhere in the world. Working as a doctor in the Armed Forces can be very rewarding and challenging. It is the advice of the authors of this guide that students who embark on medical cadetships should be committed to a career in the Services after graduation, and not simply addressing the funding of their course. The Forces recruit during the early years of the medical degree course and offer familiarisation visits for interested students. Contact details for each Service are given in the Further Information section at the end of the book.

Elective funding

Students who organise themselves well in advance can often get enough funding to pay for some (if not all) of the cost of their elective. You should have a wonderful time wherever you go, but it is so much nicer if you know you haven't paid for it all yourself. Depending on where you want to go and what you will be studying, there are numerous grants, research awards, sponsorships, and bursaries available (the BMA holds a list of organisations to whom you can apply for funds). Some will be open for all UK students to apply for, and other funds will be distributed locally. Most awards and grants are given in exchange for some sort of project report or research work.

Graduate students

Tuition fees

Fees for graduate students or self-funding students on standard courses will vary from institution to institution (see later). Some charge the standard £1125 per year, whereas others charge more for the preclinical stage of the course and more again for the clinical stage, so it is important to bear this in mind before applying and check with each medical school. Graduates who have received support from public funds for their first degree are not entitled to receive any mandatory or discretionary funding from their LEA, and would therefore be liable to pay the full cost of tuition throughout the course. The MSC has been calling on medical schools to limit the amount of fees payable by graduates to the standard £1125, but there is no guarantee of success. In response to campaigns by the MSC, the Government has introduced concessions for graduate medical students on the 4-year accelerated degree courses or GEP. Tuition fees are paid by the Department of Health in years 2, 3, and 4 of the course, and fees are payable by the students in year 1 only. The MSC is trying to persuade the Government to extend this scheme to graduate entrants on any medical degree course.

Scottish students studying on an accelerated course in the UK do not receive NHS tuition fee and bursary support in years 2–4, and are treated as though they were graduate students on a standard course – that is, means-tested maintenance loans and tuition fees.

Living costs

Graduate medical students are entitled to apply to the Student Loans Company for help with their living costs. The maximum loan available in 2003/2004 for students outside London was £4000 and for those in London it was £4930 – 25% of the loan is means tested and will depend largely upon your personal/spousal income. These figures are revised annually. Graduates on accelerated courses can apply for funding to the NHS bursary scheme in years 2, 3, and 4 of the course. Under-25s are subject to a parental means test if they apply for a bursary, and this limits its availability. The MSC is pressing for this criterion to be relaxed. Graduates on standard courses will be able to apply to the NHS bursary from year 5 onwards.

Scottish students

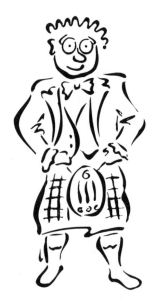

Arrangements for Scottish students vary according to whether they are studying in Scotland or elsewhere in the UK. The Student Awards Agency for Scotland (SAAS) is the body that deals with student support in Scotland (see Further information).

Tuition fees

Currently students studying at Scottish universities do not have to make a contribution to tuition fees. The Scottish Executive has set up a graduate endowment scheme whereby graduates will contribute a sum of around £2030 after they have left university (2002/2003 entrant figures). The funds raised will be used to support future students. Repayment of the endowment begins after you start earning more than £10 000 per year (in your house job). The "St Andrew's anomaly", where the preclinical students go on to do clinical studies elsewhere (usually Manchester), and therefore which funding scheme they fit into, is yet to be settled.

Living costs

The living support package you will receive differs according to whether you are classed as a young or a mature student. The Scottish Executive has introduced non-repayable maintenance grants of up to £2050 per year for students from families on low incomes and mature students with children. Maintenance loans from the Student Loans Company are also available.

Scottish students studying elsewhere in the UK

The funding for students studying outside Scotland is quite similar to that of other UK students. Your entitlement to tuition fee support is parental income assessed (up to £1100 for 2002/2003). Where there is a contribution to be deducted from the tuition fee support, the SAAS will pay the remainder.

Living costs support comes from student loans, which are the same as in the rest of the UK. There is an additional "Young Students Outside Scotland Bursary" which is available for students from families with an income below £18 400. Mature students may apply for additional grants towards the cost of child care.

Support in the fifth year and beyond

All Scottish students, regardless of their place of study, can claim an income-assessed NHS bursary and free tuition. You will also have access to a non-income-assessed student loan, repayable once your income has reached a set level, currently around £10 000 pa

The final balance...

Irrespective of your personal circumstances, studying medicine means undertaking a serious financial commitment. In common with many other students, you will have to face up to some debt and financial worries. By accepting this reality and planning before you start as to how your tuition fees, parents' contribution, bank overdraft, student loan, and bank loans will fit together over the years, you will come to terms with it better. You can find information about funding in our Further Information section. Make sure your acquaintance with debt is on your own terms. Do not avoid dealing with tough money questions and do not adopt a head-in-the-sand approach to your finances. If you anticipate difficulties during the course, take advice from the Students Union welfare services, the university, and your bank. Don't leave it too late to take action – there are very few miracle workers, and the people who are there to help are more likely to be helpful if they are given time. This talk of poverty and debt is depressing, but remember these two things.

- Debt is now a fact of life for students, and the vast majority survive and free themselves from it!
- Medical students are better placed than most to pay off their debts at the end of the day, with excellent employment prospects and job security.

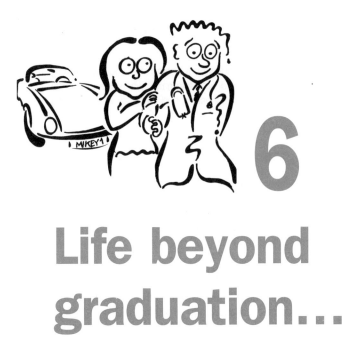

6

Life beyond graduation...

"The education of the doctor which goes on after he has his degree is, after all, the most important part of his education."

John Shaw Billings (1838–1913)

The early years

Graduating or qualifying from medical school does not in itself, allow you to practise medicine: first you must register with the GMC. Initially, registration with the Council is only provisional, but you can call yourself Doctor. To register fully, newly qualified doctors are required to complete 12 months of paid work as a house officer. This has traditionally consisted of a 6-month post in medicine and a 6-month post in surgery. However, many hospital trusts, in partnership with the postgraduate deanery, also offer a limited number of 1-year posts which consist of two 3- or 4-month units of medicine and surgery and then a further two 3-month units or one 4-month unit in other specialties such as paediatrics, general practice, accident and emergency, or psychiatry.

The ability to tailor your future career during your early working life should increase when reforms to junior doctor training are introduced in 2005. The push to modernise medical careers will introduce an integrated 2-year programme after graduation called the **foundation programme** and shorter training times to full specialisation as a GP or a consultant. Details of the foundation programme are still being finalised but a key aim is to ensure better supervision, clear educational and training outcomes, and career mentoring and advice in the first 2 years of working.

Regardless of these changes all house officer posts must be approved by the GMC for the experience to count towards full registration. At the end of your first year of working, if you can demonstrate that the minimum competencies have been achieved, you can apply for full GMC registration. Free hospital accommodation is provided for your job because the GMC believes that the right type of experience is only gained if you are resident, so don't worry if your jobs are in parts of the country that you didn't choose: there will be accommodation provided. More information about the PRHO year can be found in the BMA document *First House Job*, revised in August 2002.

Applying for your first job

Most areas operate some sort of matching scheme in the final (or penultimate) year, which is normally coordinated by the postgraduate deanery in conjunction with your medical school. At the time of writing two or three postgraduate deaneries are considering offering regional matching schemes, and a matching scheme has covered all of Scotland for some time. A house officer job-matching scheme does what it suggests – it matches prospective house officers to house officer posts. Some schemes are open to medics from any UK medical school, and some are open only to the university's own students. Some cover only the posts in the university teaching hospitals, and some cover all the hospitals in the region. Normally, the school that sends students to a hospital for clinical experience will supply the same hospital with its new house officers, but some schemes include posts that are many miles away. If you are clear that you want to work in a particular part of the country, it might be worth finding out about the matching scheme.

The advantage of matching schemes is that some of the work needed to find a job is done for you and you will be placed only in university-approved jobs. The downside is that some schemes give you little notice of where your first house job will be or leave you feeling alienated from the process. Some medical schools produce too few graduates to fill all the regional posts and some produce too many, but for the foreseeable future medics have good prospects of getting work. If you cannot get a house job in the particular town or city where you would like to work, don't worry. During the training years you can apply for jobs elsewhere in the country (and abroad). Hospitals in Australasia, for example, recruit UK doctors for short-term posts.

The BMA also provides on its website an interactive house jobs guide for members. The guide has information from hospital trusts as well as from junior doctors actually working in the trust. Having a look at this guide when you reach years 4 and 5 of medical school may prove helpful.

As arrangements may change by the time you graduate, you should take an active role in considering where you would like to live after graduation and what type of post you would like to do, well before you reach your final year at medical school.

Life as the house dog

The year as a house surgeon and physician is often the toughest in a medical career. There is much to do and learn, and sometimes providing a service to patients and your employer is at the cost of your continuing education. Current reforms aim to redress this balance and ensure that a core set of doctoring skills are gained by all house officers in the future. Be under no illusions that you are at the bottom of the medical hierarchy. Demands from your patients, your colleagues, and your bosses can be overpowering. Hours of work are long (50+ per week); however, changes to European law coming into effect in 2005 mean that the situation is slowly improving. Working intensively at night or weekends (on-call) can be exhausting.

As a house officer you will be responsible for taking histories from new patients, organising tests, following up consultants' instructions, and helping at outpatient clinics and with theatre sessions. However, there are controls and ways of reducing the strains upon you. There will probably be times when you are fed up and may want to quit medicine. Some do, but the vast majority stay on. You will become more confident, more able to cope, and the work will eventually become more interesting (and challenging).

Beyond the house officer year

After you have completed your first year in hospital and have received registration from the GMC, you can begin to follow the path you want. This has traditionally been in senior house officer posts through basic specialist training and, later, in specialist or GP registrar posts. If you have a strong idea about what specialty you want to practise in or you know you want to become a GP, then you can begin to take the appropriate path in the second year of the **foundation programme** and continue through the new **training grades**. Don't worry if you don't know which branch of medicine you want to be in now or even, for that matter, during the first few years after graduation. Many junior doctors don't decide on their final career until well into their postgraduate training and a core element of Government reform is to ensure that career advice is more readily available. The three main areas of practice are general practice, hospital medicine, and surgery. The BMA is working with the Government on ensuring that changes to junior doctor training and structures to specialisation do not disadvantage future generations of doctors and that they dovetail with existing professional outcomes.

A career in general practice

General practice is changing significantly, both as a result of changes to training pathways and because of the new contract negotiated for GPs between the BMA and Government. Many GPs will continue to be self-employed doctors who provide general medical services to patients for a Primary Care Trust, although there is also the ability to work as a paid employee in the same way as consultants are employed by Hospital Trusts. GPs usually work in small, relatively autonomous business partnerships with other GPs. The most common route to becoming a principal is to do 3 years' training as a GP registrar. This is divided into 2 years of hospital posts (in specialties such as general medicine, general surgery, A&E, obstetrics, geriatrics, or psychiatry) and 1 year working as a "trainee" in general practice. Most doctors training to enter general practice follow vocational training schemes in which the particular posts that they will rotate through are preplanned from the outset. By the time the most recent entrants to medical school graduate, it is anticipated that a greater percentage of GPs will be employees rather than independent contractors.

A career in hospital medicine or surgery

In order to become a hospital consultant, junior doctors normally rotate through 2 or 3 years of SHO jobs in medical or surgical specialties. After this, and once their choice of specialty is clear, they spend between 4 and 5 years studying in registrar posts. There are specialist registrar "rotations" that allow a doctor to prearrange 3 or 4 years of training in different hospital posts. When this training is completed satisfactorily, a Certificate of Completion of Specialist Training (CCST) is issued and the doctor can apply for consultant posts.

Similar to those for GPs, the future training paths and conditions of service for hospital doctors are also undergoing change. The BMA has agreed a new contract for consultants and there is discussion of a Certificate of Specialist Training (CST) that could be awarded for shorter periods of time served in the training grades. The BMA is opposed to the introduction of a CST and continues to discuss alternative options with the Government.

Other career paths

General practice and hospital posts provide the greatest number of jobs for doctors in the health service, but there are many other career paths. Many doctors work in public health medicine, as medical academics, as researchers for pharmaceutical companies, for the Armed Forces, and in private medicine. A great strength of practising as a doctor is the range of experience you can find in work. Flexible training is becoming more common and part-time posts are numerous. Many doctors have more than one string to their bow, and it is not uncommon, for example, for a doctor to mix private work or part-time work with their main NHS job. Putting together a portfolio career as a

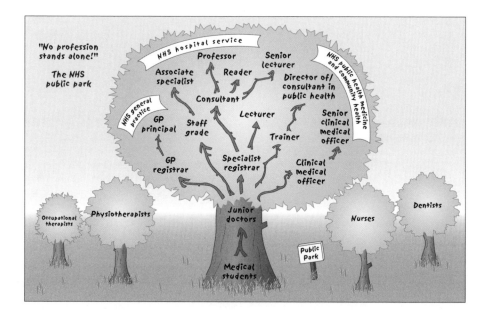

doctor is possible. A consultant might add some medical journalism and legal work in courts as an expert witness to their weekly duties as a hospital specialist; a director of public health might do voluntary medical work with a charity; or a GP might work part time with a local rugby club. The diagram on the previous page shows a simplified path of career options in medicine for doctors in the UK. There are many options open to those seeking a career in medicine. The medical career structure is outlined in the tree diagram and gives an indication of the huge variety of choices available.

Continuing medical education

Don't think that studying is over once you have graduated from medical school! The GMC's view that undergraduate medical education is just the first step toward lifelong learning means that doctors must continue to study to some extent throughout their working lives and are expected to keep their skills and knowledge up to date. The GMC has introduced a system of formal reassessment for all doctors on its register – **revalidation**. Many skills and much knowledge will be acquired "on the job", but most career paths require some formal qualifications and exams will have to be passed to retain registration with the GMC. The Royal Colleges are responsible for medical education and, for many specialties, you will need to pass membership exams to get on in your career. In other specialties, diplomas and Royal College membership exams are encouraged to supplement the minimum standards required. The introduction of revalidation and establishment of the Postgraduate Medical Education Board, which oversees all exams and diplomas offered through the Royal Colleges, will allow transparency in ongoing educational requirements across the entire profession.

Part 2
The A–Z of UK
medical schools

How to use Part 2

Numerous factors influence which medical schools suit you most and which ones you may decide to apply for. In this chapter, we have summarised a number of important areas that we think you should take into consideration before making a decision. Each medical school chapter in the following section has been deliberately divided into three sections (Education, Welfare, Sports and Social) to make it easier for you to compare different schools. A snapshot of key information for all schools can also be found at Mikey's quick compare table on page 273.

Education 📕

Although all students need to reach the same standard by the time they graduate, courses at different medical schools can vary considerably in the way this is achieved. More often than not the courses on offer are subject to change, and many of us at medical school are on different courses from those outlined in the original prospectus. Don't, whatever you do, get bogged down in the details of individual courses. You'll just get confused. However, it may be worthwhile considering the following areas.

Teaching

There are two broad teaching methods, either of which may be used on their own in some schools or combined to offer a mix of the two. "Traditional" teaching relies heavily on lectures and practicals, with a large portion of the week devoted to didactic teaching where students are in lecture theatres for long periods.

Problem-based learning (PBL) is the more recent approach, and usually has fewer timetabled commitments. Commonly, students work in small groups and discuss patient case studies, from which they form study agendas for the coming week. Students then work through their own study objectives, which are supplemented with laboratory sessions, such as pathology and anatomy in the preclinical years, and maybe attendance at outpatient clinics in the clinical years. With the PBL approach, it is essential that students, and their groups, sustain a significant amount of self-motivation.

The structure of courses also varies considerably. Some medical schools maintain the traditional preclinical/clinical divide with core science subjects, such as anatomy, biochemistry, pharmacology, and pathology taught in the early years, and speciality-based clinical subjects, such as obstetrics and gynaecology, paediatrics, and surgery taught in the later years. Other medical schools choose a system-based approach and combine both core sciences and clinical experience in all years. Between these two extremes there is all number of shades of grey and it is worth developing an idea of which style you feel you would enjoy the most.

Anatomy teaching has also seen many changes in recent years, and in some medical schools the dissection of cadavers by students has been replaced, partly or fully, with demonstration sections (or prosections) dissected by staff before class. This is often less gruesome and does not necessitate students "getting their hands wet". However, some students prefer the "hands on" approach both in and out of dissection.

Assessment

The type of assessment varies significantly between schools. Commonly used methods include multiple choice question papers (sometimes negatively marked), essay papers, short answer questions, computer examinations, literature review papers, case studies, and papers which require candidates to match questions to answers…as well as many more. Some schools have final exams in the penultimate year and others have finals at the end of the last year. Increasingly a number of schools are choosing to place a greater amount of emphasis on continuous assessment, which reduces the impact of finals at the end of the course.

When choosing which medical schools to apply for, decide whether you would prefer exams and assessments spread out during the years and the course, or whether you would prefer to take cumulative exams once everything has had a chance to fit into place. Either way, you still have to learn it all!

Intercalated degrees

This is where medical students can obtain a Bachelor of Science (BSc), Bachelor of Art (DA), or Bachelor of Medical Science (BMedSci) degree for undertaking an extra year of study (although some can be done within the "normal" 5-year course), once they have completed at least 2 years of their medical training. These degrees can be undertaken in a variety of subjects related to medicine and provide an opportunity for students to pursue further study in an area in which they are interested. UK medical schools take a variety of approaches to intercalated degrees. In some (although this approach is gradually disappearing) the extra degree is open only to the academic high-flyers; some offer courses to almost any medical student, and at others it is compulsory. If you anticipate being interested in some extra in-depth research leading to a qualification or if you think you might like to follow an academic or teaching career, then think about this before you apply. Many medical schools also allow students to study for the extra degree within other faculties of the university or at other institutions.

Special study modules (SSM) and electives

Schools devote markedly different portions of the course to studying areas of special interest (SSMs) and to overseas work placements (electives). Although there is an accepted minimum provision, it is worth considering this when choosing your medical school. Some medical schools will allow 2–4-week SSMs in more diverse subjects such as history of medicine, medicine and art, and modern languages, and certain schools allow students to take one or more SSMs abroad in addition to their elective period. The vast majority of UK medical schools offer students an opportunity to spend a longer part of the course (around 2 months), known as the elective, anywhere in the world to experience medicine in a foreign healthcare setting. The exact nature of these placements varies slightly between schools. However, wherever you choose to study, these placements are seen as one of the highlights of medical school life.

Welfare

Student support

Pastoral support systems should be in place at all universities and all students should be allocated a personal tutor or "Director of Studies". However standards of support tend to vary markedly and it is well worth asking existing medical students when you are attending the open days about the provision and success of such schemes. Some universities will provide support through the medical faculty as well as via the main campus, and a friendly, approachable and understanding medical faculty can make a considerable difference to a student's experience at university – especially if it is necessary for the student to manage ill health or dependents in addition to their medical studies. Most universities have in-house counselling and advice services.

At many universities, freshers are allocated "mummy's and daddy's" (students from later years) during their first few weeks at medical school. Such schemes can be very beneficial, helping new students to settle in and providing them with support and guidance during their early years. Many students remain in touch with their "academic families" well beyond graduation.

Accommodation

The accommodation the university provides and where it is located will have an important effect on your experience of university: remember you will spend a large portion of your time there and so you want to be happy. Important questions to ask include:

- Is accommodation provided for the first year?
- Are meals provided or is the residence self-catering?
- Is it just for medics or for a range of students?
- Is the accommodation mixed?
- Is the accommodation on campus, and if not, how far away is it?
- How expensive is the accommodation for the first and subsequent years?

Placements

Most schools will send you away from the main university hospital base for some modules. The distances involved can vary significantly. Are you the type who enjoys travelling and seeing different parts of the country or would you rather stay nearer to the medical school and spend less on travel? These are important questions to consider when applying to medical schools that have a larger number of "peripheral" hospitals. Each chapter lists examples of the distance from campus of hospital placements and journey time to give you an indication of what to expect.

Sports and social ♔

Most universities organise social weekends and freshers' weeks before the start of freshers' term, and this is a great way of making friends early on. The comfort of walking into the bar on the first evening of term and recognising a friendly face from such a weekend relieves some of the initial anxiety of leaving home and making new friends.

All medical schools offer medics' sports teams. Only students studying medicine will be able to represent these clubs. As almost all medical schools are now part of larger universities you will also be able to play for the university side. However, you tend to find that most medics pride themselves on playing for the medics. The camaraderie and social life are unrivalled and a constant envy of non-medics. However, this has also led to accusations of "cliquishness". The only limit on the number of teams you can join is the amount of time that you are willing to devote. Most students wonder how medics can study during the day, train in the evenings, and play matches week in and week out: the answer is that you develop good time management skills. However, it is important to get the balance right. One beauty of medics' sports is that all skill levels are catered for, and as you progress in your medical career you may find that you take on more responsibility for your club, from organising the mundane such as kit, to the extravagant such as tours of Europe!

Other than sports teams, most medical schools have choirs, drama clubs, and even organise annual medic shows and comedy reviews. Furthermore, most schools have medical societies that organise social events and you can also get involved with MedSin events, for example Sexpression, Marrow etc. There is something for everyone! Again, in addition to the medical school clubs, there is a wealth of university social and hobby clubs, and students are always welcome to start new ones.

Tip: Do get involved, try something new, excel at something old, but most importantly, ENJOY IT!

Aberdeen

Key facts	Undergraduate
Course length	5 years
Total number of medical undergraduates	923
Applicants in 2003	1310
Interviews given in 2003	1004
Places available in 2003	185
Places available in 2004	185
Open days 2004	24 August
Entrance requirements	ABB
Mandatory subjects	Chemistry is highly desirable. General studies is not acceptable
Male:female ratio	39:61
Is an exam included in the selection process? If yes, what form does this exam take?	No
Qualification gained	MBChB

The grey colour and cold temperature of the "granite city" bear no relation to the warm and friendly atmosphere and busy social life that is Aberdeen. The age of the medical school is not reflected in the curriculum – a new integrated systems-based course, which exploits technology to its full advantage, something that was commented on when Aberdeen was rated as excellent in a recent appraisal. Everything at the medical school and teaching hospital is on a single site (20–25 minutes' walk from main campus), so you can go straight from lectures to wards. Aberdeen medics tend to work hard, play hard, and make the most out of being a large and distinct department within a university.

Education

The 5 years are split into four phases: fundamentals of medical science; principles of clinical medicine; specialist clinical practice; and professional practice. A core syllabus focusing on integrated systems for the whole class is counterbalanced with special study modules (SSMs) for the individual. Students must complete each phase before passing on to the next. The first graduates from the new course qualified in summer 2000. Students must adopt a proactive approach, and self-motivation is an important requirement. Although the course is predominantly lecture-based, there are problem-based and tutorial-based learning sessions. Some of the course is taught through self-study packages. There is a formal staff/student committee that meets regularly and a clinical staff/student committee that meets every 5 weeks to discuss the course. Different students attend each time to give a wider viewpoint.

Teaching

Aberdeen received a very high rating in the last Scottish Higher Education Funding Council Teaching Quality assessment. Problem-based teaching is partly replacing the traditional didactic approach and students experience many different learning environments, such as general practice, specialist hospital wards, lecture theatres, tutorial groups, and the Clinical Skills Centre. Anatomy is taught via dissection. Computer-assisted learning is integrated within each phase of medical training, supplementing the compulsory ward teaching and tutorials.

Assessment

Assessment is both continual and exam-based (written and clinical), with vivas for distinction and pass-fail candidates. There is no compulsory use of animals or animal material in practicals. Should you fail a degree assessment, there are three more chances by way of two vivas and a further written exam. Students are supported and encouraged should this occur.

Intercalated degrees

About one in five students do an intercalated degree (BSc) after year 3. You must have passed all your exams and not repeated a year to be considered. All intercalated students follow a core syllabus as part of their year, followed by a research project, which can be chosen by the student. Many of these projects offer a chance to participate in clinical research, and some students have had their work published in medical journals.

Special study modules and electives

All of the four phases of the course include special study modules. The final phase SSM is non-medical, offering the opportunity to study subjects such as Spanish, history of medicine, music, or sign language. During the final phase, students have a 7-week elective period, which can be spent abroad – almost anywhere in the world. This includes a short research project, which contributes towards your final degree. It is not a holiday!

Erasmus

For further information about Erasmus, please contact Dr Frank Thies, Department of Medicine & Therapeutics, Aberdeen Medical School. Email: f.thies@abdn.ac.uk.

Unlike some other degree programmes it is not feasible for medical students to undertake a prolonged period of study abroad in a foreign medical school. There is, however, an opportunity for spending at least a limited time abroad during the project-based elective in Phase IV.

Facilities

Library   Facilities are good (open 8.45 am–10 pm Monday to Thursday; 8.45 am–8 pm Friday; 9 am–10 pm Saturday; 1 pm–10 pm Sunday). Texts and journals are plentiful, as is access to MedLine. Photocopying costs about 3p/sheet, and printing 5p/sheet.

Computers   There are many computers available, with free internet and email, and plenty of printers. There are excellent computer-assisted learning packages for a variety of subjects, as well as practice exam questions. Virtually all lecture presentations are available on the internet for viewing before to ensure that note-taking is kept to a minimum and more time can be spent listening to what the lecturers are saying. There is 24-hour access to computer laboratories on the university campus and at the medical school.

Clinical skills   The clinical skills laboratory sited in the hospital grounds is equipped with up-to-date medical technology. It is used for teaching clinical skills and procedures to all medical students and many junior doctors, with timetabled access and "drop-in" sessions run by senior specialists (eye examination by an ophthalmologist, for example). These include examination skills, use of equipment, communication skills (interviewing simulated patients), and many practical procedures, for example iv access, suturing, catheterisation, defibrillation, etc. A "Harvey" cardiology patient simulator is now used to teach all students from year 2 upwards.

Welfare

Student support

There are regular staff–student liaison meetings, excellent relationships with lecturers, and the Dean is very approachable. There is a large support network should things go wrong, including academic tutors, individual advisors ("Regent Scheme"), trained counselling staff at the university, and the usual main university NUS welfare support.

Accommodation

University flats and halls accommodation are readily available for all years of study, although most people move into private accommodation after their first year. Private accommodation is in high demand and can be expensive.

Placements

The medical school is based at the Foresterhill Hospital site, so you can go straight from lectures to the wards. During the final 2 years you study at hospitals in either Inverness, Fort William, or Elgin for 5–10 weeks. Placements in Shetland and Stornoway, introduced in 2001, were oversubscribed with volunteers. GP attachments are now available throughout Scotland – most located in rural

Location of clinical placement/name of hospital	Distance away from medical school (miles)	Difficulty getting there on public transport*	Accommodation available
Royal Cornhill Hospital	1	+	No
Woolmanhill Hospital	2.5	++	No
Woodend Hospital	2.5	++	No
Dr Gray's Hospital, Elgin	70	+++	Yes
Raigmore Hospital, Inverness	106	+++	Yes

*Ease of accessibility: +, set your alarm clock early; ++, long journey; +++, car is a must

surroundings. Free accommodation is provided, as is travel at the beginning and end of the attachments.

Studying at one of the largest teaching hospitals in Europe allows Aberdeen medical students to experience all specialties on a single site. A new children's hospital is due to open on site in 2004. The learning environment is relaxed and friendly, with the medical staff rewarding you with the help you need as long as you put in the effort. Written finals are completed at the end of year 4, leaving time to earn up to £160 a week working as a student locum. Students on placements away from Aberdeen enjoy excellent teaching, social life, and free accommodation close to the hospital. The newly introduced "island" attachments involve one-to-one teaching from a consultant and provide excellent experience, especially if you are a budding surgeon. However, some students might find these placements a bit too isolated.

Sports and social 🏆

City life

The city centre is compact and lively, with most pubs and clubs within a 10-minute walk of each other and a 20-minute walk from most student halls. Aberdeen is a prosperous town. The revenue brought in by the oil industry is apparent when you look at the excellent provision of shops, pubs, and other services. However, this can make Aberdeen expensive to live in. Glasgow and Edinburgh are both easily accessible, and Aberdeen has excellent travel links.

Just a short journey from the buzzing centre is the beach, with roller coasters, an ice-rink, and a new cinema. In the other direction are the hills and the outdoors: great for walking, climbing, winter, and water sports. The northerly location means that the climate can be very cold and, although there are excellent road, rail, and air links, Aberdeen is a considerable distance from anywhere else. People from far away (UK and overseas) can get a bit homesick and find Aberdonians more hostile than they actually are – but the strong friendships you will make in Aberdeen will help you through this.

University life

As the medical school is isolated from other parts of the university, medics need to make a bit of an effort to meet non-medical students, but year 1 is normally spent in halls and this gives students an opportunity to meet others outside medicine. Most student social life tends to revolve around drinking! The medical school refectory has recently been renovated – it now includes "Costa Coffee" – great after a night out! The union runs many organised events and the Medical Society holds functions every 2–3 weeks and hosts a very popular annual ball. University societies are numerous and healthy, covering a wide range of interests: sporting, dramatic, photography, musical, outdoor, university Armed Forces units (army, navy, and RAF), intellectual, and malt whisky appreciation just to name a few. The medical school has a few societies of its own, and the annual medical revue is well supported and popular.

Sports life

The Aberdeen Medical Students Society (MedSoc) has its own rugby, football, cricket, and hockey teams, which compete against the other Scottish medical schools. MedSoc members can join an exclusive gym in town for a discounted fee of £100 per year. The main university offers a wide range of sports as varied as gliding, underwater hockey, and archery, as well as regulars such as rugby, hockey, and football. Members of all levels are given a warm welcome. There are no specific medical school facilities, but the university offers an inexpensive gym, pool, and tennis facilities, among others.

Fascinating Fact: Aberdeen has the highest pub to person ratio in Britain!

Great things about Aberdeen

- Friendly small school, with teaching hospital and medical school buildings within a single site.
- Excellent student social life, with civilised licensing laws (late opening: 3 am at the weekend).
- Easy access to the great outdoors (beach and mountains a very short distance away; skiing 45 minutes away; sailing locally).
- Patient contact from the first term of your first year!
- New clinical skills centre with lots of great teaching equipment and online resources.

Bad things about Aberdeen

- No dedicated medics' social centre on site.
- Travelling from Aberdeen often involves a long journey and living far away from home.

- Geographically isolated from the rest of the university, which means the majority of your student friends are medics – this is not helped by the different timings of exams and holidays.
- Cold in the winter – actually it's cold most of the rest of the year too!
- The people can appear cold.

Further information

College Office
College of Life Sciences and Medicine
Polwarth Building
Foresterhill
Aberdeen
AB25 2ZD
Tel: 01224 554 975
Fax: 01224 550 708
Email: f.a.galloway@abdn.ac.uk
Web: http://www.abdn.ac.uk/medicine/prospective-students

Additional application information

Average A-level requirements	• ABB in three A-levels taken at first sitting. Chemistry is highly desirable to grade B, plus at least one other from biology/human biology, mathematics or physics and one other. General studies is not acceptable
Average Scottish Higher requirements	• Five Highers at AAAAB obtained at first sitting. Two subjects from biology, maths, physics: H biology preferred over H physics in Y5
Graduate entry requirements	• 2:1 Hons
Make-up of interview panel	• Two admissions selectors with at least one clinician
Months in which interviews are held	• October–March
Proportion of overseas students	• 8%
Proportion of mature students	• 27% (based on 2004 intake)
Proportion of graduate students	• 24% (based on 2004 intake)
Faculty's view of students taking a gap year	• Acceptable
Proportion of students taking intercalated degrees	• 20%
Possibility of direct entrance to clinical phase	• No
Fees for overseas students	• £9960 pa (preclinical) and £18 570 pa (clinical)
Fees for graduates	• See Chapter 6
Ability to transfer to other medical schools	• Students can choose to study an intercalated BSc at any other university providing term dates match
Assistance for elective funding	• Many grants and other financial awards are available
Assistance for travel to attachments	• Bus travel provided to placements in Inverness
	• Travel costs can be reclaimed for periods of study outside Aberdeen
Access and hardship funds	• Apply through central university fund
Weekly rent	• £35–£50 per week
Pint of lager	• £2 (But many cheap student deals available)
Cinema	• £3–£5 depending on the night
Nightclub	• The centre of Aberdeen has a busy nightlife with something to suit everybody

Bart's and The London

Key facts	Undergraduate	Graduate
Course length	5 years	3 years 8 months
Total number of medical undergraduates	1300	40
Applicants in 2003	2000	1200
Interviews given in 2003	1120	150
Places available in 2003	268	40
Places available in 2004	268	40
Open days 2004	July	July
Entrance requirements	ABB	2:1
Mandatory subjects	Chemistry and biology	Sciences
Male:female ratio	116:155	17:23
Is an exam included in the selection process? If yes, what form does this exam take?	No	Yes, PQA
Qualification gained	MBBS	MBBS

St Bartholomew's and the Royal London Hospitals, or Bart's and The London, Medical School resulted from the merger of St Bartholomew's and The Royal London and is centred in London's East End, one of the capital city's most exciting areas. Home to a large number of ethnic groups, this area is a fascinating place to study medicine as a result of the varied needs of its communities.

St Bartholomew's is the oldest hospital in the world and is a centre of excellence for many specialist disciplines. The Royal London was the first medical school in England and will be the site of our new medical school building, to be completed in 2004. Plans are also under way to build a 1000 unit student village at the Mile End campus.

The school strives to be progressive, and the 2004 intake will be the sixth year to study the new 1999 curriculum, which has problem-based learning at its core and a greater emphasis on the integration of clinical and preclinical elements of medical training.

The combined school of St Bartholomew's and The Royal London is part of Queen Mary College, University of London (QMUL). As it was the first school to complete the merger process, all of the difficulties associated with such a transition are now a thing of the past. Indeed, it is believed by some to be one of the most innovative and forward thinking schools in the UK.

Education

The curriculum, started in 1999, is centred on the technique of problem-based learning (PBL). This approach involves a reduced number of lectures, and students are encouraged to find their own answers to clinical problems using textbooks, journals, and the internet, as well as practical experience. All students follow the same core course, and are then able to broaden their knowledge in areas of particular interest during special study modules (SSMs). The traditional preclinical/clinical divide is now less distinct, as the new course integrates basic medical, human, and clinical sciences from day one until graduation. Bart's and The London students are placed with both GPs and hospitals during the first 2 years.

Teaching

In the first 2 years of the course, teaching is systems-based, concentrating on "Systems in Health" for year 1 and "Systems in Disease" for the second. There is a mixed approach, including lectures, PBL, and workshop sessions, and all aspects of the body system, such as the cardiovascular system, are considered as an integrated whole. For the final 3 years teaching is hospital-based, with a continued emphasis on self-directed learning. Courses in communication skills (using actors and videotaping), and ethics run throughout the 5 years. Dissection is no longer part of the core course, and anatomy is taught using computer-aided learning programs, anatomical models, and predissected specimens. Those who wish to dissect may do this as an SSM. St Bartholomew's, The Royal London, The London Chest and Homerton Hospital are the home sites for clinical teaching, although as with all of the great teaching hospitals in London there are a large number of other hospitals where students have an opportunity to get an experience of different areas of medicine. These extend right out to Southend and Harlow.

The faculty at Bart's and The London is keen to respond to student feedback and a lot of time and effort is spent by both staff and students in fine tuning the curriculum. This has resulted in a course that both the staff and the students are very proud of.

Assessment

Summer exams are set for years 1–4 of the course, and with the new curriculum, "big bang" final examinations are a thing of the past. Assessment is continuous, with credit being given for performance in both tutorials and examinations. The emphasis that has been placed on student feedback has resulted in great strides being made in assessment. In particular Bart's and The London is proud of the fact that it is one of only a few medical schools in the country where the MCQ-style questions have been phased out of the assessment programme. At the end of year 5, students are assessed on their "competence to practise" as a PRHO and must pass an integrated paper and clinical exams.

Intercalated degrees

Both BSc and BMedSci courses are offered and popular courses include Experimental Pathology and Medical Science (BMedSci). Some students have studied anthropology, psychology, and even German, although this kind of choice is rare. Students can choose to stay at Queen Mary College or go to another university to study for their intercalated degree. Fees are payable for the year, but some funding is available. Allocation of places on intercalated degree courses is on a competitive basis, but all courses offered within the school will involve research-based projects and not just library-based projects.

Special study modules and electives

There is a wide variety of SSMs available, including clinical, research, complementary medicine, and journalism. It is also possible for some students to spend 3-month attachments at partner institutions in Europe. The elective lasts 2–3 months, starting after Christmas in year 5 of the course. There are some existing arrangements with institutions in other countries in Europe, and several student-led exchange programmes with institutions all around the world, which can make organising a trip more straightforward. However, students can, and have, gone almost anywhere as long as they can find themselves a supervisor.

An advantage of the Bart's and The London course are the opportunities for foreign travel. Any of the Special Study Modules, of which there are two every year, can be used as an opportunity to study abroad. Most students use one of the 4-week SSMs in the final year to study overseas in addition to their 6-week elective.

Erasmus

Bart's and The London has a long history of exchanging students within the Erasmus programme with the world famous Karolinska Institute in Stockholm. Other regular exchanges occur with the Lund as well as several other universities.

Facilities

Library There are three large libraries, one at each site. The two hospital libraries have wonderful architecture, history, and atmosphere. The library at Queen Mary College is large and can occasionally be noisy during the daytime. The availability of books is variable depending on the time of year. Libraries are open 9 am–9 pm on weekdays and 9 am–4 pm on Saturdays. The College library is also open on Sundays. In addition there are two large pathology museums at the hospitals. Unfortunately, in light of the events at Alder Hey Hospital, access to these is now severely restricted.

Computers The school is well equipped on all three sites. Computing facilities and functions are available and regularly updated. Computers are increasingly used for teaching and are available during library hours and from 10 am to 8 pm at weekends. There is also 24 hour internet access on the QMUL campus during the week and the computer rooms at the medical schools are open late.

Clinical skills   The Clinical Skills Centre at Bart's is for use by both medical and nursing students and is available to everyone in the school. In addition first-years learn clinical skills in an adapted ward at Mile End Hospital.

Welfare

Student support

On the first day of college, freshers are assigned a senior student to act as their "parent" and guide them through the first few weeks and beyond. "Parents" introduce their "children" to their friends, take them out to dinner, and offer advice on all issues, from simple things such as work to more complicated matters such as relationships. This enables a great deal of integration between students from different years. All students are allocated their own academic tutor. In addition, for personal and other problems, they have the use of a pastoral pool of sympathetic doctors and senior lecturers. The Medical and Dental Students' Association appoints a student as Welfare Officer, as does QMUL Students' Union. Counselling is available within 24 hours at QMUL and is provided by a dedicated and independent advice and counselling service. Students with mental health problems can be seen in confidence by a consultant at another teaching hospital as part of a reciprocal arrangement with another school.

Accommodation

Students at Bart's and The London can spend 2–3 years of their studies in college accommodation. New first-year students choose whether they wish to live in Queen Mary College or University of London (intercollegiate) accommodation, and whether they wish to be catered for or to cook for themselves. Most first-years live in either Dawson Hall, which is an old Bart's residence, or Floyer House at The Royal London. In the past, students have also lived in South Woodford, which was the cheapest and most social halls. However, it has become less popular as it is rather run down and a long way from Mile End. At the end of 2004, a brand new student village project will be opened on the Mile End campus. This will provide new, but rather expensive accommodation very close to lectures. Dawson Hall is a very modern facility, the main attraction of which is its beautifully set location near St Paul's in the centre of London. It is very hard to get into as a first-year student and so early applications are essential. It allows students to self-cater, as does Floyer House, which has recently been refurbished and is close to the Union. There have been some questions as to the safety of this residence set within Whitechapel. In central London, students from all colleges of the University of London live together in intercollegiate halls. These are a 30-minute tube ride away from college. With all residences, students should check whether or not rent is payable during holidays. As with all halls of residence in London the cost is relatively high. London generally is an expensive place to study and live, although there is a lot of development going on.

Most senior students live in the East End in shared houses. Almost everyone lives within walking distance of The Royal London and QM sites. Property is slightly cheaper in east London than in other parts of the capital. The Griffin Community Trust provides cheap (about £50 per week), luxurious housing in a very special development incorporating housing for the elderly, a community centre, and flats for clinical students. Student residents spend an hour or two a week with their elderly neighbours

Location of clinical placement/name of hospital	Distance away from medical school (miles)	Difficulty getting there on public transport*
Barts	2.4	+
Homerton	4.7	++
Whipps Cross	6.8	++
King George's	12	++
Southend	38.4	++

*Ease of accessibility: +, set your alarm clock early; ++, long journey

and play bingo, watch videos, or just chat. Both students and elders say how much they gain from the experience.

The important thing to remember is that Bart's and The London has a lot of relatively cheap, affordable housing located near the college. Therefore when its time to move out of halls you are able to move to a location, which will minimise the amount of money you spend on travel.

Placements

The medicine course is based at three sites: Bart's, The London, and QMUL, which are all within 3 miles of each other in the City and East End of London. They are easily accessible by tube, bicycle, and bus. The Medical Sciences department at QMUL in Mile End is where the first 2 years are based currently, although this is due to change in 2004–2005 with the building of a new medical school in Whitechapel. This site has good facilities, including the Students' Union shop, computer laboratories, and the ever popular "E1" nightclub. The final 3 years are spent in hospitals. Many of the district general hospitals used are in or close to the East End and accessible by bus or tube. Several are close enough to cycle to.

Students can expect to be sent to attachments outside the main teaching hospitals. Placements are in district general and other associated hospitals. Accommodation is provided free. Destinations include Southend-on-Sea, Chelmsford, and Harlow. GP attachments and SSMs can be arranged countrywide and worldwide.

Sports and social ♔

University life

The Medical and Dental Students' Association is thriving and provides social and sporting opportunities as well as welfare services for all. The two medical student bars at Bart's and The

London hold regular discos and theme nights. Wednesdays (after sports matches) and Fridays are the main nights for going out. A large TV screen in the bar regularly shows the main sports events. The summer ball at Bart's is popular, and there are smaller balls for freshers' week, rag week, and at Christmas.

The college prides itself on its charitable rag week. Last year medical and dental students raised over £150 000 from events including street collections, marathon running, bed-pushing, and even a fashion show. It is one of the most successful rags in the country and the biggest in London. Freshers' fortnight is equally popular and a massive effort is made to welcome new students to the college.

There are over 30 clubs and societies run by the Bart's and The London Students' Association. These offer students the chance to develop new interests, meet people, play sport, and have a good time. Among the most active societies are: the Drama Society, which stages productions every term, including the infamous Christmas show, and travels to the Edinburgh Festival; the Asian Society, which organises the famous international fashion show, celebrating the diversity of culture within the school, annually raising many thousands for charity; and the Music Society, which includes the choir, orchestra, brass groups, and several bands. QMUL has more clubs and societies if there are not enough at the medical school, or if you have a particular interest not catered for.

Student social life revolves around the Association/Union buildings at both Bart's and The London. The Medical Student President is head of the Medical and Dental Students' Association and takes a sabbatical year from his or her studies solely to represent and protect the interests of the medical and dental student community. The newly refurbished Association building at The London, and the bar at Bart's, are for use by medics, dentists, and their guests. In The London Association building there is a café-bar and bookshop. The official Association magazine, *M.A.D.*, comes out at least twice a term and reports on social, sporting, and other events. A large Students' Union is also available at the QMUL Mile End campus.

Sports life

The Bart's and The London Students' Association clubs cater for nearly all sporting interests and the majority welcome beginners. There is an off-site sports ground and there are swimming pools at both Bart's and The London Hospital. There are gyms at Bart's and QMUL College and squash, tennis, and badminton courts are available at QMUL. Bart's and The London have an enthusiastic rowing club, based on the River Lea, and hockey, water polo, women's football, and rugby have been successful in recent years. The cricket club is legendary, with strong first and second teams which win titles most years.

Fascinating Fact: David Burckett St Laurent, a current fourth-year at Bart's and The London, became the youngest ever person to walk to the North pole in 2003 to raise money for charity.

61

Great things about Bart's and The London €

- An innovative curriculum and teaching, as well as enthusiastic and approachable staff.
- All students and visitors agree that we are a friendly community with a close-knit atmosphere; students tend to have friends from all years, rather than just their own.
- Reasonable rents for shared houses, considering that we are in the centre of London, and everyone lives close to each other.
- There are good year-round events, and the Union bar opens with regular late licences.
- Diverse area, with a wide range of things to do and cultures to experience – the East End is very trendy, with new bars and restaurants opening all the time; the *Evening Standard* recently nominated Tower Hamlets as London's sexiest borough!

Bad things about Bart's and The London

- Local areas – we are surrounded by very deprived communities and, although this means good clinical experience and pathology subject matter, it can be a bit depressing; at times, it is necessary to be wary, as students have been assaulted.
- Travelling – there is some travelling between sites required, and the rush hour lasts for hours, although congestion charging has meant very fast bus links.
- Little interaction with non-medical and dental students in the past resulted in some rivalry between the medics and QMUL students; however, most of these issues have been fully worked out now.
- London is such a massive place that it can take some time to feel at home in its vastness.
- Expense – living and studying in London is more expensive than elsewhere; this is the biggest draw back to studying at Bart's and The London, as it is for any London medical school.

Further information

Admissions Office
Bart's and The London School of Medicine and Dentistry
Turner Street
London E1 2AD
Tel: 020 7377 7611
Fax: 020 7377 7612
Email: medicaladmissions@qmul.ac.uk
Web: http://www.smd.qmul.ac.uk

Additional application information

Average A-level requirements	• ABB. Chemistry and biology at AS-level, plus another science at A-level
Average Scottish Higher requirements	• AAAAB with Advanced Highers in chemistry/biology at grade B
Graduate entry requirements	• 2:1 in a science based degree
Make-up of interview panel	• Three, usually comprising clinician, basic medical scientist, and clinical student
Months in which interviews are held	• November–March
Proportion of overseas students	• 9%
Proportion of mature students	• 25%
Proportion of graduate students	• 25%
Faculty's view of students taking a gap year	• Acceptable
Proportion of students taking intercalated degrees	• 60%
Possibility of direct entrance to clinical phase	• No
Fees for overseas students	• £12 000–£22 000
Fees for graduates	• See Chapter 6
Ability to transfer to other medical schools	• Possible in cases of extenuating circumstances after completing the first two years successfully
Assistance for elective funding	• No bursaries available
Assistance for travel to attachments	• None
Access and hardship funds	• College administers access-type funds
Weekly rent	• Halls £65–£100; private £60 upwards (average £80)
Pint of lager	• £1.70 Union bar; £1.80–£2.50 city pub
Cinema	• £3.80 upwards
Nightclub	• £4 upwards

Belfast

Key facts	Premedical	Undergraduate
Course length	6 years	5 years
Total number of medical undergraduates		910
Applicants in 2003		595
Interviews given in 2003		23 (consisting mainly of graduates, plus a few others)
Places available in 2003	5	180
Places available in 2004	5	180
Open days 2004		Early September
Entrance requirements for 2004	Irish Leaving Certificate or Scottish Highers (A-levels not accepted)	AAA + A in AS
Mandatory subjects	Applications are considered on an individual basis	Chemistry to A-level and biology to at least AS-level
Male:female ratio		39:61
Is an exam included in the selection process? If yes, what form does this exam take?	No	No
Qualification gained, eg BmedSci BMBS	MB BCh BAO	

Queen's University of Belfast provides a relaxed and informal integrated medical course. Ninety per cent of the students come from Ireland (both north and south), and a strong emphasis is placed on social life and enjoyment. The school also sits in a perfect position to access Belfast's nightlife, arguably the best in the UK. Queen's is the only medical school where it is not illegal to enjoy a good night's craic! Discussions are taking place to increase the size of the medical school, with more undergraduate places. However, as yet there have been no plans to implement a graduate accelerated course.

Education 🔖

A traditional preclinical/clinical divide is less evident on the new course, and teaching combines a problem-based approach with more traditional lectures from year 1. Clinical skills are taught from year 1 in hospitals, in general practice, and in a clinical skills centre. Each year is divided into two semesters, and the trend is for year groups to be divided into smaller groups for teaching. In years 1 and 2 students learn the basic science of medicine with an integrated systems approach. The sociological and psychological aspects of medical practice are emphasised and special study modules are taken. In year 3 the systems are taught again, but with an emphasis on mechanisms of disease. More time is spent in hospital attachments at this stage, and year 4 students spend all their time on the wards in hospital attachments or in general practice. The final year is a consolidation process with no new subjects.

Teaching

Teaching in years 1 and 2 consists of lectures, tutorials, laboratory practicals, and meeting patients, both on the wards and in general practice. There is a mixture of demonstration, dissection, and prosection for teaching, and animal tissue is used in physiology. During years 1 and 2 only half a day a week is spent on the wards. In year 3 blocks of specialty-based integrated teaching are supplemented by pathology lectures and tutorials. Teaching is very much self-directed, with the clinical aspects being taught on the wards. Years 4 and 5 are completely ward-based. Computers and clinical skills are used for training throughout the course. Ward group sizes in teaching hospitals tend to vary, but efforts are made to keep the numbers as small as possible to benefit both the patients and the students. The friendliness of the staff and their willingness to teach varies from ward to ward. Most, however, are willing to help in true Northern Irish fashion.

Assessment

Years 1 and 2 have specific subject exams at the end of each semester with an overall recap exam at the end of year 2. Year 3 is examined by coursework throughout the year and end of semester clinical exams. In year 4 exams are at the end of each 8-week block. If needed, resit examinations start in the second week of August and last for a week or two. However, most students try to give exams their best so as to maximise the holiday period. Procedure cards need to be completed as part of A&E medicine, anaesthetics, fractures, and obstetrics and gynaecology. Final examinations take place in two parts: the written examinations take place in September at the start of the final year, and the clinical examinations are held at the end of the final year, although there is a possibility that this will change. During the final year the overseas elective, a clinical project, refresher clinical placements, and a clinical apprenticeship are completed.

Intercalated degrees

Between 5% and 10% of students take a BSc during their course, usually after years 2 or 3. Science degrees are available in anatomy, biochemistry, physiology, microbiology, pharmacology, and medical genetics. It is possible to study degree subjects that are not available at Queen's by making arrangements with another institution. However, approval for this has to be sought from the Dean. If there is competition for places, previous results in the respective subject will often determine entry. Students from Northern Ireland may be eligible for Local Education Authority (LEA) or bursary funding for the year.

Special study modules and electives

During the summer vacation between years 3 and 4, students have the option to arrange elective "pupilships" for a period of 4–6 weeks at a hospital in the UK. This is optional and the student takes responsibility for organising the placement. In the final year students are encouraged to spend their elective period overseas. Students must also carry out a 6-week clinical project, either overseas or at Queen's, followed by the production of a project report of between 7000 and 10 000 words.

Erasmus

QUB is attempting to expand its Erasmus programme at present and is currently canvassing students for their opinions and interests. Opportunities already exist for students who wish to study at medical schools in Switzerland, Spain, Germany, and Norway. Almost all students will use the overseas elective as an opportunity to see new shores and spread their horizons.

Facilities

Library   There are two main medical libraries, the largest in the Royal Victoria Hospital (RVH) and a smaller one in the Belfast City Hospital (BCH). They both have online catalogues, with access to networked journals, MedLine, and other databases. They close at 9.30 pm on weekdays and 12.30 pm on Saturdays. Study space is available at the Belfast City Hospital and at the Medical Biology Centre (MBC) outside the library opening hours. The MBC houses an anatomy study room with access to a library of microscope slides and computerised anatomical guides. Each peripheral attachment has some library provision, although this varies from hospital to hospital, and medical students are more than welcome to use the libraries and facilities of the wider QUB campus. All library books are catalogued in a computerised searchable database.

Computers   The RVH and the MBC each have computer facilities available for medical students. When the IT suites and other libraries of QUB are taken into account, computer provision is usually more than adequate although, just before an essay deadline or exam session, things can tend to clog up. All computers are fully networked, although certain applications for medicine can only be accessed from the MBC or RVH.

Clinical skills   The Clinical Skills Education Centre (CSEC) provides teaching on practical medicine and affords students a chance to do some "hands-on" learning. Through a mix of simulated patients (often drama students from QUB), life-like models and tuition from practising clinicians, students are taught various clinical skills, which are later assessed in the CSEC at end of semester examinations. Students have the opportunity to practise clinical skills at the CSEC and also on their clinical attachments.

Welfare

Student support

Each medical student is allocated to a consultant, known as their Faculty Tutor, whose role is to help with any problems. Staff in the faculty office are friendly and approachable, as is the current Dean. The Students' Union also has a counselling service and provides access to academic and financial advice. Rails, ramps, and lifts are available in many areas for disabled access. A recent minding scheme has been started (called MAFIA) whereby each student is allocated a "godfather" who looks after the personal aspects of student life.

Accommodation

There is a place in university halls for every student who wants one. The rooms tend to be warm and comfortable, with good food but thin walls. Catered rooms cost between £50 and £65 per week and self-catering rooms £45–£61.50 per week, inclusive of heat and light. They are about half a mile from the university, but can mean a trek if an early lecture has been scheduled for the RVH. Private accommodation is available closer to faculty, although there can be no guarantees as to price or quality. Generally a room in a private house will cost between £150 and £200 per month with the average rent being £170. The Lisburn Road area of Belfast is extremely popular with medical students, as it is close to the MBC, the BCH, and the RVH.

Placements

In years 1 and 2 most of the teaching takes place on campus in the MBC and the BCH. These are about a 15–20-minute walk from the halls of residence. Other lectures and clinical work take place at the RVH, a 35–40-minute walk from the halls. However, a free bus runs from the BCH to the RVH every 15 minutes. From year 3 onwards students receive teaching in the RVH, and clinical attachments may be throughout the Province. The RVH recently underwent renovation, the result of which is a brand new hospital, with great teaching facilities. In addition, hospitals and GP practices outside central Belfast are used from year 3 onwards. Hospital and GP accommodation is free, and the furthest one might travel would be about 80 miles from Belfast. However, with the notoriously poor transport infrastructure, it may take a disproportionate amount of time to travel a short distance. This means spending part of the week in a peripheral hospital for a portion of the academic year – which can make a change from Belfast but can also seriously affect extracurricular activities.

Sports and social 🏆

City life

Belfast is a lively welcoming city with much to offer visitors. The student area is only a mile away from the city centre but surprisingly self-contained – many students only rarely venture out of the mainly

Location of clinical placement/name of hospital	Distance away from medical school (miles)	Difficulty getting there on public transport*	Accommodation available
Belfast City Hospital	0	+	No
Royal Victoria Hospital	1	+	No
Musgrave Park Hospital	2	++	No
The Ulster Hospital	5.5	+++	No
Altnagelvin	72	+++	Yes

*Ease of accessibility: +, set your alarm clock early; ++, long journey; +++, car is a must

student Malone and Stranmillis areas to Belfast's more upmarket city centre. All tastes are catered for in Belfast with a wide range of pubs, cafés, and clubs, and the Students' Union hosts one of the biggest club nights in Ireland on a weekly basis. Those with a more cultural orientation will find themselves amply provided for by the range of drama, music, and art available to students. The Queen's Film Theatre is an award-winning art-house cinema located within the university campus.

Although you may have your hands full coping with what Belfast has to offer, it is easy to travel further afield. Dublin is just over 2 hours away by train, and it is a must to visit the Giant's Causeway, the Mourne Mountains, and the Fermanagh Lakes, all of which are within 90 minutes of Belfast.

University life

Student life in Belfast is largely centred around the Students' Union, a few other student venues and the Physical Education centre. For medical students the Belfast Medical Students' Association (BMSA) runs an active programme of social events, providing medicine with a social cohesion that is the envy of every other faculty. Every year the BMSA runs a freshers' three-legged pub crawl, a mystery tour, a fancy dress party, the annual faculty ball, a staff–student dinner, and regular discos attended by all years. Year 4 runs its own annual revue – tasteless but entertaining – and a medical charity called SWOT, which raises money by organising blood pressure clinics, street collections, a fashion show (with local TV celebrities), and pub quizzes. Queen's also has an active MedSIN group. The Sudents' Union has three bars and runs regular discos, balls, and concerts. Like most universities, there is likely to be a society for whatever you want to do.

Sports life

There are many sports clubs at Queen's, most of which compete in the Province's leagues. Near the university there are playing fields, tennis courts, and a boat club. The Queen's Physical Education

Centre has everything you need to keep fit. It is beside the university, well equipped, and costs 70p to get in if you are a student.

Fascinating fact: The Belfast Medical Students' Association is the oldest and largest student society at Queen's.

Great things about Queen's

- An updated curriculum so that students gain clinical experience from year 1 with small group teaching.
- Queen's has an international reputation for trauma care, cardiology, and ophthalmology.
- Belfast is compact as a capital city but has everything you need.
- The social life – fortnightly events – are organised by the Belfast Medical Students Association (BMSA) so inter-year relations are good.
- Relaxed and informal atmosphere.

Bad things about Queen's

- The weather – there is no danger of students blowing their allowance on suntan lotion.
- The weekends tend to be quiet – many students go home at the weekend, particularly in year 1.
- The siting of the main medical library means that at night students can only get to it by car.
- The ready availability of the "Ulster Fry" pushes your waistband.
- The high number of students on some attachments.

Further information

Admissions Office
The Queen's University of Belfast
University Road
Belfast
BT7 1NN
Tel: 028 9033 5081
Fax: 028 9024 7895
Email: admissions@qub.ac.uk
Web: http://www.qub.ac.uk

Dean's Office
Tel: 02890 245 133 ext 3477
Fax: 02890 330 571

Additional application information

Average A-level requirements	• AAA chemistry to A-level and biology to at least AS-level
Average Scottish Higher requirements	• Considered individually
Graduate entry requirements	• Minimum 2:1 in a science based degree
Make-up of interview panel	• Three – Admissions Tutor plus two members of academic staff
Months in which interviews are held	• February/March
Proportion of overseas students	• 7%
Proportion of mature students	• 3%
Proportion of graduate students	• 3%
Faculty's view of students taking a gap year	• Acceptable
Proportion of students taking intercalated degrees	• 10%
Possibility of direct entrance to clinical phase	• No. There is a formal partnership with the International Medical College in Kuala Lumpur
Fees for overseas students	• £8415 (premedical); £10 160 pa (preclinical), and £18 725 pa (clinical)
Fees for graduates	• £1125
Ability to transfer to other medical schools	• Contact admissions directly for advice
Assistance for elective funding	• Various grant scheme and faculty bequests are available
Assistance for travel to attachments	• Available through the Education and Library Boards for students entitled to a grant
Access and hardship funds	• Some university funds and bequests are available but amounts are small
Weekly rent	• Halls: single room catered £65, single room self-catered £54.50 (£65.50 en suite)
	• Private £35–£50
Pint of lager	• Union bar £1.60; city centre pub £2.00
Cinema	• £2.50–£4.00
Nightclub	• £2–£10

Birmingham

Key facts	Undergraduate	Graduate
Course length	5 years	4 years
Total number of medical undergraduates	1700	43
Applicants in 2003	1614	999
Interviews given in 2003	1100	120
Places available in 2003	346	40
Places available in 2004	346	40
Open days 2004	23/24 April and 18 September	
Entrance requirements	AAB	2:1 (minimum)
Mandatory subjects	Chemistry (biology at least to AS-level)	Life science degree Chemistry at grade C
Male:female ratio	2:3	3:4
Is an exam included in the selection process? If yes, what form does this exam take?	No	No
Qualification gained, eg BmedSci BMBS	MBChB	MBChB

Birmingham Medical School is on the northwest edge of the main University of Birmingham campus, just a few miles from the city centre. It is a large provincial medical school, with a great diversity of students, a well-established modern course and clinical experience introduced from the second week of study. The admissions tutors believe strongly that doctors should be well-rounded individuals and not just dedicated bookworms. This is well reflected in the mix of students and the lively social scene at the medical school, which ranges from sport, drama, and politics, to partying. From the first week as freshers until the final year dinner, held a week before graduation, students at Birmingham can expect to both work hard and play hard.

Education

The first two years of the medical course follow a systems-based approach. Regular patient contact in general practice begins within a few weeks of starting the course and full-time hospital teaching commences in year 3 for both medicine and surgery. Pathology and epidemiology are also taught during year 3. Years 4 and 5 involve rotating through specialties such as paediatrics, oncology, and orthopaedics, in addition to senior medicine and surgery. Students on the graduate entry course (see Chapter 4), which started in September 2003, will study the basic sciences in their first year. In year 2 they will study a course similar to the standard year 3, and will be fully integrated with the rest of the medics for years 3 and 4.

Teaching

Preclinical teaching involves lectures and follow-up tutorials incorporating problem-based learning exercises. There is no dissection at Birmingham, but we have excellent models to work with in a specially designed laboratory. Histology teaching is all done by video and accompanied by colour course booklets – there is no straining down microscopes for Birmingham medics! Hospital teaching combines bedside teaching, observation, small group teaching sessions, and participation in clinics and procedures.

Assessment

Modular examinations take place after Christmas and in the summer term. Exams can consist of multiple choice question papers (MCQs) and short and long answer papers, and some in-course assessment is a feature of most modules. First-years have to pass a practical exam in basic life support, and in the later years clinical subjects are examined by MCQs and Objective Structured Clinical Examinations (OSCEs). Students are expected to pass every module in order to proceed to the next year. First-years also have to pass a practical exam in basic life support. Viva examinations may be held for borderline pass or Honours candidates.

Intercalated degrees

An increasing number of students at Birmingham are choosing to intercalate, typically after year 2, for an Honours Bachelor Degree in Medical Science (BMedSc), and after years 3 or 4 for a Masters in Medical Science (MMedSc). This can be in the biological sciences, such as physiology, pharmacology, neuroscience, or pathology, and involves a laboratory-based research project (and a chance to publish!). Alternatively, you can do an integrated health science, such as public health, ethics and law, behavioural science, or history of medicine. The history of medicine is particularly popular and we have an internationally renowned unit based in the medical school.

Special study modules and electives

Eight special study modules (SSMs) are completed during the course. There is a choice of many topics, with new ones starting all the time. In the clinical years, these become more self-directed and clinically orientated, and are commonly conducted outside the medical school. However, currently only the elective can be taken abroad. Electives are taken at the end of year 4 and normally last 2 months. They provide an opportunity to travel and experience medicine anywhere in the world.

Erasmus

Currently there are no overseas travel opportunities aside from the elective, but the medical faculty are very keen to start some.

Facilities

Library   The library is conveniently situated within the medical school and has an extensive range of medical textbooks and journals. It has plenty of quiet study areas and computer facilities with access to MedLine, the internet, and library catalogues. It also has extensive photocopying facilities. During term time it is open from 8.45 am to 9 pm Monday to Thursday, until 7 pm on Fridays, and from 10 am to 6 pm at weekends.

Computers   The computer cluster is very futuristic – a vision in blue and steel! There is a mixture of Apple Macs and iMacs (about 100) on the east side, and about 100 PCs on the west side. The computer cluster is open 24 hours, and you are automatically credited with 1000 free laser print credits, although printing is unlikely to remain free. Every computer is online and allows full access to computer-assisted learning packages that supplement the course. Computer facilities are also available in general practices, teaching hospitals, and all of the district general hospitals (DGH) that host student teaching.

Welfare

Student support

The pastoral care at Birmingham is provided by a network of approachable student tutors and is excellent. There is also an effective student-run Curriculum and Welfare Committee that is respected by staff. Students are placed into families, with three to four students from each year group. A social event is held each term by the tutor group, meaning that you will always know a few people in other years.

Accommodation

Accepting a conditional offer from Birmingham guarantees a place in university halls or flats for year 1. All university accommodation is within 2–3 miles of the campus and most are within walking distance. The Vale is a complex of several halls and flats and has the greatest overall capacity. The style of accommodation ranges from large traditional halls to flats with en-suite bathrooms. All halls have good security and excellent committees and social events. There is an excess of private rented accommodation available at reasonable prices in Selly Oak, a centre for students and just minutes away from campus. Selly Park, Harborne, and even Edgbaston (which is, in parts, very posh) are also very popular.

Location of clinical placement/name of hospital	Distance away from medical school (miles)	Difficulty getting there on public transport*	Accommodation available
Queen Elizabeth Hospital	1	+	No
Heartlands Hospital	12	++	No
City Hospital	12	++	No
Good Hope Hospital	15	++	No
Wolverhampton Hospital	20	+++	No

*Ease of accessibility: +, set your alarm clock early; ++, long journey; +++, car is a must

Placements

Situated in the suburb of Edgbaston, the university is just a couple of miles from the city centre. The medical school (which adjoins the Queen Elizabeth teaching hospital) is found at the west end of a refreshingly spacious and green campus. It has benefited from the recent refurbishment and upgrading of lecture theatres, tutorial rooms, computer facilities, and student common rooms. There are four large teaching hospitals in the city of Birmingham, as well as specialist hospitals and numerous district general hospitals. Medics at Birmingham will have very few long-term attachments outside the West Midlands, and the majority of placements are within commuting distance of student accommodation. Don't be fooled by the relatively short mileage between the medical school and hospitals – the 12 miles to Heartlands can take anywhere from 15 to over 45 minutes.

During years 1–4, groups of four students attend a general practice once every fortnight. This offers a valuable early introduction to patient contact and clinical skills. The family attachment scheme is another community-based project that takes place in year 2. From year 3 onwards, students attend hospital placements full time for most of the year, with occasional teaching sessions in the medical school.

Sports and social 🏆

City life

Birmingham is a cosmopolitan city. All the big-name stores and designer shops can be found in the city centre, most of them in the new Bullring complex – a mecca for those who list "shopping" as one of their hobbies. The city has a vast selection of restaurants, serving everything from Alaska cod to zabaglione, plus all the curry you could ever wish for. Birmingham boasts a vibrant nightlife, ranging from the quintessential student night to jazz clubs and trendy bars. There are plenty of theatres, and the national indoor arena, NEC, and Symphony Hall regularly play host to major international acts and are literally on our doorstep! The city and surrounding area are well served by public transport. There is in fact a train station just next to the medical school that connects to Birmingham New Street station, and from there to just about anywhere. Birmingham International Airport is also accessible directly by train. More rural locations, such as the Malverns, Stratford upon Avon, and the Black Country, are all easily reached.

University life

Not only is medicine the largest faculty in the university, but related courses such as medical science, physiotherapy, dentistry, and nursing are also based in and around the medical school. There is considerable social integration between all these students and between different year groups. An enthusiastic medical society and final-year dinner committee ensure that there is always something happening. As the medical school is located on campus, medics can easily retain involvement in university activities and social events and thus experience the best of both worlds.

The medical society organises the renowned freshers' conference, regular pub crawls, wine tasting, curry quizzes, theatre trips, ski trips, and a post-exam annual camping extravaganza to the Gower. Calendar events held in the medical school include the musical, a very funny comedy revue, and the glamorous final-year fashion show. Many events are held in city centre venues, which are easily accessible by public transport and cheap for a taxi home. The medical school magazine, *QMM*, was revived a few years ago and affords an opportunity to put pen to paper. There is an active surgical society for those people who think that they might be budding surgeons, and MedSIN and Marrow can be found making a difference to the lives of others. The Birmingham University Guild of Students (BUGS) houses the usual complement of bars, clubs, and pool tables, as well as a society for every imaginable interest, from Rag committees to cocktail parties!

Sports life

The university has an excellent reputation for sport. The athletics union runs an impressive range of different sporting clubs. The medics also run large clubs for hockey, rugby, football, netball, cricket, tennis, and basketball. Medics rugby, hockey, and netball teams have all been national medical school champions in recent years. The clubs are friendly and well supported (especially in post-game celebrations) and cater for all ranges of ability, from absolute beginners to international players.

> **Fascinating Fact:** The first trials of the contraceptive pill outside the USA were based at Birmingham Medical School.

Great things about Birmingham

- Fully integrated course with early clinical experience keeps your interest levels up.
- Excellent relations between years and with other degree students.
- IT facilities and support are very good.

- The new medical student welfare system is first-rate.
- Good range of hospitals used during attachments.

Bad things about Birmingham

- Having to do proper research during the elective (spoiling the holiday).
- The eternal traffic jam on the Bristol Road and M6.
- The wait for exam results, particularly in early years, can be rather long.
- The security guards are very diligent, so, if you forget your ID card, they won't let you into the medical school.
- Expensive and unvaried food at the medical school canteen.

Further information

Professor C J Lote
Admissions Officer/Tutor
Medical School
University of Birmingham
Edgbaston
Birmingham B15 2TT
Tel: 0121 414 6888
Fax: 0121 414 7159
Email: c.j.lote@bham.ac.uk, admissions@bham.ac.uk
Prospectus requests: prospectus@bham.ac.uk
Web: http://www.medweb.bham.ac.uk

Open days: 23/24 April 2004.

Additional application information

Average A-level requirements	• Grades AAB to include chemistry and one of biology, physics or maths. Biology to AS-level if not A-level
Average Scottish Higher requirements	• AAAAB in chemistry, biology, physics, maths and English and 2 Advanced Higher (general studies not accepted)
Graduate entry requirements	• 2:1 or better in a life sciences degree
Make-up of interview panel	• Admissions Tutor, one or two representatives from the medical community
Months in which interviews are held	• October–March
Proportion of overseas students	• 7.02%
Proportion of mature students	• 6%
Proportion of graduate students	• 6%
Faculty's view of students taking a gap year	• No problem provided there are plans to use the year constructively
Proportion of students taking intercalated degrees	• 20%
Possibility of direct entrance to clinical phase	• No
Fees for overseas students	• £9900 pa (preclinical) £19 100 pa (clinical)
Fees for graduates	• £1125 pa LEA pays year 1. Year 5 paid by NHS
Ability to transfer to other medical schools	• Transfers are rare, but possible and are usually as a result of personal circumstances or family problems
Assistance for elective funding	• There are a few intraschool trusts and the Medical School Office keeps an exhaustive record of all local trusts that medical students can apply to; however a lot of people have to fund themselves
Assistance for travel to attachments	• This is fairly limited; it usually works out as about £5 a week for placements over ten miles away
Access and hardship funds	• Some grants and bursaries are available
Weekly rent	• Private £45–£50
Pint of lager	• £1.90
Cinema	• £3.30
Nightclub	• £2–£10

Birmingham

Brighton and Sussex Medical School

Key facts	Undergraduate
Course length	5 years
Total number of medical undergraduates	135
Applicants in 2003	1000
Interviews given in 2003	500
Places available in 2003	128
Places available in 2004	128
Open days 2004	22 June, 8 September
Entrance requirements	ABB
Mandatory subjects	Biology & chemistry to AS-level, one to A-level
Male:female ratio	42:58
Is an exam included in the selection process? If yes, what form does this exam take?	No
Qualification gained	BMBS

The Universities of Brighton and Sussex were successful in their bid to host a medical school as part of the Government's expansion plans for training doctors and the first cohort of students began their studies in September 2003. Brighton and Sussex Medical School (BSMS) is a partnership between the Universities of Brighton and Sussex and the new Brighton and Sussex University Hospitals NHS Trust.

Students are members of both universities, and enjoy access to the academic and recreational facilities of each. The two universities have biomedical research interests recognised by grade 5 research ratings. Sussex has one of England's largest Biological Sciences Schools, while Brighton has extensive experience in education and training of health professionals including postgraduate doctors, nurses, midwives, pharmacists, physiotherapists, and medical laboratory scientists.

The two universities have adjacent campuses at Falmer, with fast rail and road links to central Brighton. Brighton, newly elevated to city status, has a vibrant social scene to which the universities' students (over 10% of the population) make a prominent contribution. The campuses also have direct pedestrian access into the planned new South Downs National Park, long recognised as an area of outstanding natural beauty.

Education

In the first two years academic and clinical studies are based in new facilities at the Falmer campuses. Direct experience of working with patients takes place from the first term. Clinical experience at this stage is in Primary Care and Community Medicine settings, and you carry out two individual family studies – in year 1 with a family looking after a new baby and in year 2 with a family including a dependent requiring continuing care. Students also experience medical practice in some hospital settings, including visits to a busy A&E unit. Allied to this is development of clinical, communication skills, and the study of functioning of the human body using a system-based approach. Systems modules include the core material and are centred around weekly Clinical Symposia that employ a problem-based learning approach. They also include student-selected options that allow you to explore selected topics in greater depth.

During years 3–5 you gain progressively more experience in clinical contexts, and the requirement to integrate clinical experience with an understanding of the underlying clinical and social sciences and public health issues continues. Students keep individual clinical skills and personal development portfolios that are used to assess progress. Studies are based at the new Medical Education Centre at the Royal Sussex County Hospital, Brighton. Year 5 is essentially an apprenticeship year to prepare you for your postgraduate year as a Preregistration House Officer (PRHO).

Teaching

A wide range of teaching methods are employed, with the emphasis on the small group academic and clinical teaching possible in a small and personal medical school. Individual patient studies, in which clinical findings and treatment are related to the principles of the underlying clinical and social sciences, develop an understanding of the practice of medicine.

The BSMS degree also gives insight into the astonishing pace of development of understanding in the biomedical sciences and you can gain experience in medical research as a member of a BSMS, Brighton or Sussex research team through your year 4 *Individual Research Project*.

Assessment

BSMS uses a variety of assessment methods to continually monitor student progress throughout the course. Individual modules are assessed (assessment includes MCQs, extended matching questions and short answer questions) at the end of each 10-week period to ensure that the module objectives have been met. There are also practical assessments that test for good clinical and communication skills throughout the course. Each student receives a personal portfolio where they record all the work that they do in the year, for example module essays, presentations, computer skills, etc – these portfolios are regularly viewed by personal tutors and also contribute to part of the assessment. Pass grades must be achieved in all aspects of the course to progress to the next stage; however, there are opportunities to retake any element that you do not succeed in passing at the first attempt.

The main formal assessments are at the end of year 3 and year 5.

Intercalated degrees

Intercalated BSc degrees are offered subject to performance. The degree is done between years 3 and 4 of the BMBS degree and subjects that are available to study include biomedical sciences, biological sciences, biochemistry, molecular genetics, molecular medicine, and neuroscience.

SSMs and electives

Throughout the BSMS programme students get the opportunity to study special areas of interest in more detail. These may be medically or scientifically based but there is also the option to choose a topic relating to the arts or humanities, for example. Student selected components (SSCs) may be either laboratory-, hospital- or seminar-based and are led by a tutor or a clinician with an expert knowledge of the field.

Electives are undertaken during the first 8 weeks of year 4. BSMS has relationships with a number of countries and a choice of placements will be available. As we are currently the first intakes to the medical school, it is hard to say any more about the elective module as we have no older students to question about their experiences.

Facilities

Library   As a student at BSMS you have access to both the University of Sussex and Brighton libraries as well as the Medical Postgraduate library. All libraries offer student study areas, IT suites, and extended access hours.

In addition to these facilities, a new medical library is currently being built at the Royal Sussex County Hospital, which has been designed to cater for all students and staff needs.

Computers   Both the University of Brighton and Sussex libraries are well equipped with PCs. In addition there are other large clusters on campus where students can use a range of software applications.

The BSMS also has its own brand new computer suite, which offers access only to medical students within the medical school itself.

Clinical skills　　There is a new medical education centre at Royal Sussex County Hospital Brighton and a state of the art dissection room and IT suite.

Welfare

Student support

BSMS is very aware of the physical, emotional and intellectual demands placed on medical students and so has placed a lot of emphasis on student support. Throughout the degree, students are supported by both academic and personal tutors who encourage you to go to them with any problems or difficulties that you may be experiencing both within and outside of the course. During year 5, link tutors are added to the support group to provide advice and guidance to students during their clinical attachment when they are away from the main medical school.

Other sources of help include chaplaincies, childcare facilities, disability and learning support, financial support, health services, personal counselling, sexual health, welfare advice, and careers advice.

Accommodation

On campus accommodation is guaranteed in year 1 as long as you meet the deadline for handing in the housing application form. Accommodation is allocated on either the Sussex site or the Falmer (Brighton) site. Single, double, and family rooms are all available on campus and prices are varied so there is accommodation to suit everyone. Halls are all of a good standard and all the rooms on the Brighton site are en suite! As all accommodation offered to first-year medics is on campus, a sense of community arises very quickly after the beginning of term. Medics are mixed in with non-medics, which provides medical students with a good way of meeting other students studying at both Brighton and Sussex university.

In years 2,3, and 4, students are required to find their own accommodation in and around Brighton. There are loads of suitable places to rent and many areas are particularly student friendly. If you find that you are having difficulties finding somewhere to rent, then the universities accommodation services are always on hand to offer help and guidance.

During year 5, accommodation will be provided close to the regional centre hospital that you are based in.

Placements

In years 3 and 4 students undertake a range of clinical attachments, mainly at the Royal Sussex County Hospital but extending into other trust and primary care settings.

In year 5 students undertake clinical attachments in two different regional locations chosen from the list below. All hospitals are in the areas surrounding Brighton and link tutors are attached to each

Location of clinical placement/name of hospital	Distance away from medical school (miles)	Difficulty getting there on public transport*	Accommodation available
Hastings, The Conquest Hospital	40	++	Not determined
Haywards Heath, Princess Royal Hospital	15	++	Not determined
Tunbridge wells, Kent and Sussex Hospital	30	++	Not determined
Worthing, Worthing District General Hospital	10	+	Not determined
Brighton, Royal Sussex County Hospital	2	+	Not determined

*Ease of accessibility: +, set your alarm clock early; ++, long journey

hospital making sure that you are supported during your year away from the university. There is also PRHO shadowing.

Sports and social 🏆

City life

Brighton recently gained city status and has long been known as "London by the sea". The new city has a relaxed but lively atmosphere and offers something for everyone.

It boasts over 200 pubs and bars and has a reputation for being the clubbing capital of the south coast. There are dozens of clubs to choose from, some of which open out directly onto the beach and attract big name DJs.

The city also offers a range of restaurants and shops, which include the arty North Laine boutiques to the more well known high street stores, such as those found in the Churchill Square shopping complex.

You'll never be lost for something to do in Brighton and if you ever feel like escaping city life you've got the beach and South Downs Way on your doorstep!

University life

As a student at BSMS you will be part of a small and friendly medical school in a supportive environment. The medical school is brand new and as a result you will have access to "state of the art" facilities such as the dissection room and IT suite.

In year 1 you will be based and will spend most of your time in the medical school itself, situated on the Falmer site, University of Sussex. However, you will also spend time on the University of Brighton campus as well as afternoons in primary and secondary care settings.

As a student at BSMS you can make use of both universities' facilities. Sussex is a campus-based university and you will find everything you need on site, from a Post Office to a cocktail bar. The campus has many "plus points" including its surroundings (South Downs Way) and sense of community. However, if you ever feel like getting away from it all, Brighton town centre is only a short train journey away.

Sports life

The good thing about BSMS is that, as we are spread over two universities, we get two universities' worth of sports facilities. You also can choose to join either the Sussex sports teams or the Brighton sports teams, depending on which one you think you will do best in. Once you have decided to join one sports team, you're not committed to that university and can still join the sports teams for the other one.

The Falmer campus has sports halls, fitness rooms, dance studios, squash and tennis courts, soccer and rugby pitches, floodlit artificial turf pitches, sauna and solarium, and a lifestyle studio offering a sports injury clinic, sports massage, reflexology, and beauty therapy.

There are sports clubs in almost every area you can imagine, including a number of watersport clubs that take advantage of Brighton's seaside location. If there isn't a club that interests you and you would like one, then all you need to do is get together a group of about five students and approach the Union for funding – more often than not you will be given some help to set up your club.

Currently there are no specific medical school sports clubs owing to the fact that we are the first intake. However, we are trying at the moment to set up a medical society and hope that through this, and after a few more students have joined BSMS, we can develop some medic specific teams to compete against both the rest of the university and other medical schools.

Great things about BSMS

- BSMS is a small medical school so you will be part of a friendly and supportive environment.
- As a student at BSMS you will be part of a new medical school with all its brand new facilities.
- Staff, both at the medical school and within the clinical settings, are very enthusiastic.
- At BSMS we practise full dissection in a brand new dissection room.
- Brighton is a great place to live!

Bad things about BSMS

- Coffee queues at the local coffee shop between lecture breaks.
- Parking!
- Getting back to campus after a night out.

- Relatively expensive especially compared to some northern towns/universities.
- You seem to spend loads more time in lectures than other students at the university!

Further information

For further information about the Brighton and Sussex Medical School and its curriculum, see its website: www.bsms.ac.uk.

For general information on studying at the Universities of Brighton and Sussex visit their websites; www.brighton.ac.uk and www.sussex.ac.uk or contact the BSMS admissions office:
BSMS Admissions
University of Brighton
Mithras House
Brighton
BN2 4AT
Tel: 01273 600900
Answerphone: 01273 642825
Fax: 01273 642828
Email: admissions@brighton.ac.uk
Web addresses: www.brighton.ac.uk, www.sussex.ac.uk

Additional application information

Average A-level requirements	• ABB, biology & chemistry to AS-level, one to A-level
Average Scottish Higher requirements	• ABB at Advanced Higher, must include chemistry or biology, both to Higher level
Graduate entry requirements	• 2:1 Hons preferably with biology and chemistry to at least AS-level
Make-up of interview panel	• Three panel members, comprising a member of BSMS faculty, a GP, and a third member who may be a hospital consultant, a junior doctor, or a member of another health profession
Months in which interviews are held	• November and February
Proportion of overseas students	• 0%
Proportion of mature students	• 28%
Proportion of graduate students	• 23%
Faculty's view of students taking a gap year	• Students are welcome to apply to BSMS during year 13 for deferred entry or during the gap year itself. They must, however, be available for interview
Proportion of students taking intercalated degrees	• Provision made for intercalated year, but no students will reach this stage until 2006
Possibility of direct entrance to clinical phase	• No
Fees for overseas students	• N/A
Fees for graduates	• £1125
Ability to transfer to other medical schools	• Check directly with the medical school
Assistance for electives funding	• New school, no information at present
Assistance for travel to attachments	• New school, no information at present
Access and hardship funds	• Yes all students eligible to "access to learning funds" currently through the Welfare department at Sussex
Weekly rent	• £50 upward (private)
Pint of lager	• £2
Cinema	• £2 upward
Nightclub	• £3 upward

Bristol

Key facts	Premedical	Undergraduate	Graduate
Course length	6 years	5 years	4 years
Total number of medical undergraduates		c 1000	
Applicants in 2003	240	1852	Information unavailable
Interviews given in 2003	35	694	194
Places available in 2003	10	217	19
Places available in 2004	10	217	19
Open days 2004	24 June		
Entrance requirements	2:1 or AAB	AAB	2:1 BSc
Mandatory subjects	Non-science	Chemistry & one other science subject	Biomedical science
Male:female ratio	1:2	1:2	1:2
Is an exam included in the selection process? If yes, what form does this exam take?	No	No	No
Qualification gained	MBChB		

Bristol is one of the old red-brick universities complimented by a very modern and dynamic course. As well as a close-knit medical school, there are numerous opportunities to enjoy friendships within the wider student body. The city centre provides an excellent and reasonably compact environment in which to work and play, and the university itself has an excellent reputation, producing high-quality research and supporting good teaching. Bristol also offers a premedical year to a small number of students each year, in which the teaching is with predental students and provided by departments in the Faculty of Science. In addition, a 4-year fast-track medical course for graduates opened in October 2003. Currently there are just 19 places and the course is only available to Honours graduates in biosciences (see Chapter 4).

Education

Bristol introduced an integrated curriculum in 1995. The integrated course consists of three phases. Phase I, lasting two terms, acts as an introductory period and provides a basic understanding of the human body and the mechanisms of health and disease (molecular and cellular basis of medicine). Phase I also has a human basis of medicine component, where students learn medical sociology, ethics, and epidemiology. This is mainly taught in the School of Medical Sciences. Phase II lasts until the end of year 3 and consists of mixed clinical and theory-based systems-orientated teaching. Phase III includes teaching and clinical experience of specialty subjects (such as paediatrics, obstetrics, and gynaecology). In addition, phase III includes the elective period and senior clinical attachments in medicine and surgery. Clinical contact begins in general practices in year 1, and the first hospital attachment is in year 2. During phases II and III the whole year group is regularly brought together in Bristol for lectures and tutorial teaching.

Teaching

Early-phase teaching consists mainly of lectures and practicals, supplemented by small group tutorials and some self-directed learning. (No live animals are used in practicals, although occasionally some tissue, such as crab legs and guinea-pig ileum, is used in experiments.) Topographical anatomy is taught by young medical demonstrators using cadaveric prosections. Students have the opportunity to do a short dissection project in anatomy in their second year. Anatomy is a popular and rewarding element of the medical degree course at Bristol.

Assessment

Regular assessments are conducted throughout the course. Many clinical attachments include projects or the preparation and delivery of a case presentation, whereas science teaching carries associated tutorial and practical work. There are usually exams at the end of each year, although continuous assessment contributes to the final-year mark. There are particularly important exams at the end of year 3, in addition to finals at the end of year 5.

Intercalated degrees

Undertaking a BSc is a popular option, with about 30% of students opting to intercalate. The school positively encourages students to intercalate, usually after year 2, but it is possible to do so after year 3. Students may choose a conventional science subject, such as biochemistry or pathology, although recently programmes such as bioethics have been introduced. The Honours year gives students an opportunity to try some "real" science in the form of a potentially publishable original research project, as opposed to the rather structured medical course.

Student selected components and electives

SSCs are an important part of the new curriculum from year 1 onwards, allowing students to pursue subjects of special interest. Elective time is currently 8 weeks at the beginning of year 5 and most students opt to travel abroad.

Erasmus

During year 3 students can choose to study abroad for a period of 18 weeks. Locations include Paris, Bordeaux, Vienna, Oslo, and Finland. In addition some SSCs (student selected components) can be taken overseas, although the student is responsible for finding a supervisor considered satisfactory by the central coordinator in Bristol.

Facilities

Library The medical library is open until 9 pm on weekdays (5 pm or 6 pm during the long vacation) and on Saturdays. The main library has longer opening hours. Popular textbooks are available from the medical library on a short loan basis. MedLine, Embase, and other databases are on open access on library computers, as are email and internet connections, which are also available in the halls of residence.

Computers Computers are available in the medical school (including the library) and in the main library. There are a number of 24-hour open-access rooms dotted around the university. Computer-assisted learning packages are available in the medical library. Other terminals support internet access, email, word processing, etc. Information technology is supposed to be an integral part of the new course, but the quality of computing facilities is variable.

Clinical skills All the teaching centres have facilities, though the primary site is in one of the main teaching hospitals in Bristol, the Bristol Royal Infirmary. In year 2 adult life support is taught and students are examined and certified. The clinical skills laboratory is also used to teach venepuncture to second-year students. As students progress through the course, other clinical procedures, such as intubation, may be learnt here or in the medical academies (see Placements).

Welfare

Student support

There is a personal tutor scheme in operation and it normally works well, the quality of the scheme depending on the tutor (and the tutee). However, most students find a member of staff with whom they get on well and from whom they can seek help. The faculty tends to be supportive, provided they are informed of problems before they get out of hand. There is a staff–student liaison committee, but input does not often translate into immediate action. The university and the Students' Union both have counselling services. Access for students with disabilities may be difficult because of the layout of the university (on a steep hill). The secretary of Galenicals (the medical students' society) is also there to voice student opinions and views to the medical faculty.

Accommodation

Most first-years are accommodated in university halls of residence. These tend to be comfortable enough and provide an excellent opportunity to bond with other freshers (medics and non-medics)

Location of clinical placement/name of hospital	Distance away from medical school (miles)	Difficulty getting there on public transport*	Accommodation available
BRI, Bristol	0	+	No
Frenchay/Southmead Hospitals, Bristol	8	+	No
Bath	13	++	Yes
Weston Super-Mare	26	++	Yes
Taunton	50	+++	Yes

*Ease of accessibility: +, set your alarm clock early; ++, long journey; +++, car is a must

at the numerous organised events or in the hall bars. The main group of halls is located at a 30–40-minute walk from the university precinct. It is possible to apply to stay in halls after year 1, but most people move into university flats/houses or into accommodation in the private sector. Weekly rents vary, but most students pay between £55 and £70. It is usual to pay rent over the summer and the scrum for houses starts quite early in the year. The accommodation office provides some help, but a lot depends on individual initiative.

Placements

The first two years are spent mainly around the university campus in central Bristol. When you begin clinical specialty attachments you can be placed at one of the main Bristol hospitals or anywhere within a 50-mile radius of Bristol. Attachments start in year 3. Medical academies are being established in Taunton, Bath, Cheltenham, Swindon, and Gloucester. The concept of an academy is a group of teachers and students (up to 80) focused on medical school activities and with equivalent resources to the home university. Students will usually spend 6 months at each academy, and during the 3 years, half the time will be located in academies within Bristol. General practice attachments are also spread across the south-west. Accommodation is provided wherever it is essential for students to be away from Bristol. However, although some help is given with travel expenses, travel to and from these attachments can be an extra expense (especially if you want to come back every weekend). A car is a huge bonus, but trains or buses serve all the hospital attachments, but not all the general practice ones.

Sports and social 🏆

City life

Bristol has a lot to offer both as a university and as a city. The university is a research-orientated institution with an excellent reputation but also provides good teaching. The city is just brilliant fun.

Mainstream attractions abound and there is plenty of "alternative" entertainment for those who want it. It is still reasonably safe (at least in the areas frequented by students), provided appropriate precautions are taken. It is certainly no worse than most other cities in this respect.

The city centre is reasonably compact and packed with things to attract all comers. The countryside (and the attractions of the West Country and Wales) is not far away. Students tend to congregate in the areas just around the university, such as Clifton. However, there is a shift towards areas a little further away, which offer cheaper rents. Clifton is the most affluent part of Bristol, offering pleasant cafés and bijou shops. Shopping, theatre, museum and music lovers will all find something to their taste. There are plenty of pubs, restaurants, clubs, cinemas (including three "arthouse" cinemas), plenty of parks and green spaces, and all the other things you would associate with a vibrant city like Bristol.

University life

Entertainment abounds in Bristol – sometimes there seems to be too much choice! A number of big acts play at the university and at other venues throughout the city. There is a huge range of societies to join at the Union. Halls and Galenicals lay on a range of entertainment, organise a number of sports teams, and represent students' views on a variety of committees. There are two revues for medics to take part in. The preclinical revue tends to be a rather drunken and disorganised affair, but the clinical one is a more organised and moderate event that runs for four nights in the Union theatre. Galenicals organises a lot of events for medics and has its own bar, which students from all year groups use.

Sports life

The university has good outdoor facilities, tennis centre, and a brand new indoor centre within the campus. Wednesday afternoons are usually free for sport, and there are teams at all levels in most sports. There are a number of medics' teams (including the infamous Women's Football Team) organised through Galenicals, which tend to be a bit less competitive than the university teams. They have a considerable social component (and alcohol consumption, too!).

Fascinating fact: Jonathan Webb, former England Rugby Union player, qualified as a doctor at Bristol.

Great things about Bristol

- Friendly and close-knit.
- The generally high standard of teaching and the high quality of clinical experience, especially in peripheral hospitals.
- The city of Bristol itself, with its huge range of bars, restaurants and attractions.
- The opportunity to mix with plenty of non-medics and medics from other year groups.
- A modern, clinical course in which student feedback is valued.

Bad things about Bristol

- The rather conservative nature of the university in terms of atmosphere and politics.
- The financial costs (high rents; long distance attachments in clinical years; expensive bus fares).
- Walking up all those steep hills (Bristol is one big hill)!
- Feedback on exams you have just taken can sometimes be a bit limited.
- Huge annual scramble for accommodation at a reasonable price.

Further information

Admissions Office
University of Bristol
Senate House
Tyndall Avenue
Bristol
BS8 1TH
Tel: 0117 928 7679
Fax: 0117 925 1424
Email: admissions@bristol.ac.uk
Web: http://www.medici.bris.ac.uk

Prospectus requests: 24-hour answerphone service 0117 928 9000 ext 4021 or 0117 925 0177.

Additional application information

Average A-level requirements	• AAB, including chemistry
Average Scottish Higher requirements	• AAAAA
Graduate entry requirements	• 2:1 in biomedical science
Make-up of interview panel	• Clinicians, pre-clinicians, GPs & non-clinical personnel
Months in which interviews are held	• November–March
Proportion of overseas students	• 5%
Proportion of mature students	• 6%
Proportion of graduate students	• 6%
Faculty's view of students taking a gap year	• Acceptable
Proportion of students taking intercalated degrees	• 30%
Possibility of direct entrance to clinical phase	• No
Fees for overseas students	• £11 000 pa (preclinical) £20 500 pa (clinical)
Fees for graduate students	• £1125
Ability to transfer to other medical schools	• Possible, at any stage, assessed on a personal level. Not many do transfer, but help will be given to students having a genuine need to transfer
Assistance for elective funding	• Many bursaries available including Medical Elective Bursary, MedChi Prize, Medical/Dental prize, and external bursary funding from, for example, Wellcome Trust
Assistance for travel to attachments	• Return travel paid for plus accommodation provided
Access and hardship funds	• Available through Student Union, in line with other university arrangements
Weekly rent	• £65
Pint of lager	• £2
Cinema	• £4
Nightclub	• £3

Cambridge

Key facts	Undergraduate	Graduate
Course length	5¼–6 years	4 years
Total number of medical undergraduates	c.1950	80
Applicants in 2003	1190	245
Interviews given in 2003	Nearly all	75
Places available in 2003	278	20
Places available in 2004	278	20
Open days 2004	June/July and September – college open days 1 and 2 July – university open days	15 June
Entrance requirements	AAA at A-level	2:1 degree
Mandatory subjects	AS-level: chemistry and two of maths, physics and biology A-level: one of chemistry, biology, maths, physics	Any discipline
Male:female ratio	46:54	44:56
Is an exam included in the selection process?	Yes	
If yes, what form does this exam take?	BMAT	
Qualification gained	BA and then MB/BChir	MB/BChir

Standard Cambridge undergraduate medical teaching involves two courses: a traditional preclinical course and a clinical course. The 3-year preclinical course is a science degree in its own right: intercalation is compulsory unless you are already a graduate, and there is a strong emphasis on research. The clinical course continues that emphasis, and it is possible to intercalate an MPhil or a PhD. Until now the clinical course has been very intense and only 2.25 years long with finals in December, but from 2005 onwards it will be a 3-year course.

All Cambridge students are members of a college, and this is the focus of social life for most preclinical students. Despite the intensity of the course there is ample opportunity for extracurricular activities, not just within the colleges but also in the university and within the city itself.

Cambridge also has a 4-year graduate-entry course, which mixes elements from the standard preclinical and clinical courses with dedicated teaching; it is open to UK/EU graduates of any discipline. Graduate entry to the standard course is also possible, and is the only option for non UK/EU graduate students.

Education ▌

Cambridge has two separate courses which you need to complete for a medical degree. Preclinical medicine is taught by the Faculty of Biology, and clinical by the School of Clinical Medicine.

All preclinical students read for a BA. For the first 2 years students study Part IA and Part IB of Medical and Veterinary Sciences. The main subjects (biochemistry, pharmacology, etc) count both towards requirements for entry into clinical school ("2nd MB" subjects) and your BA. Some options are only examined for the BA, and some compulsory courses (one with a small amount of clinical contact) only count towards the 2nd MB.

Year 3 (Part II) of the BA is compulsory, unless you already have a degree (in which case you receive your BA after 2 years then go on to clinical study). It is possible to study any Part II that will accept you, such as law or social sciences, but in practice most students are strongly encouraged to study a science subject. In most of these you will spend some time on a project, usually with the chance to carry out some original research.

The preclinical course will give you a very strong grounding in the medical sciences and a BA, plus the chance to study a wide range of subjects in your Part II. Patient contact is minimal until you start clinical.

Interviews for the clinical course take place in the February prior to entry. Roughly half the students in most years stay on; the others go mainly to Oxford or London, but some go to other compatible courses, such as at Edinburgh. If you complete the 2nd MB you will get a place somewhere, although staying on at Cambridge is not guaranteed, but in most years everyone who applies to stay on is accepted. If you apply to the Cambridge clinical course after preclinical elsewhere, it is essential to complete a BA or BSc as well as equivalents of the 2nd MB before starting.

Currently the clinical course is intensive, lasting only 27 months. Most of the work is ward- or clinic-based and students are expected to be active in seeking out patients to clerk. From 2005 there will be a completely new clinical course taking 3 years.

Students on the 4-year graduate-entry course are admitted to the Clinical School from the start and do not study for a BA. During the first 2 years they combine studying for the 2nd MB with dedicated clinical teaching based at the West Suffolk Hospital, 30 miles east of Cambridge. For year 3 they join the standard clinical course, then return to dedicated teaching for year 4.

Teaching

The preclinical teaching is mainly in a traditional lecture and compulsory practical (eg anatomy dissection) format. The lecturers often teach on their research area, and can go into considerable detail. The main occasions when students discuss and ask questions about the lectures are supervisions. These small group tutorials (usually two to three students) are led by someone either involved with or familiar with the course, for example, a lecturer, or a PhD or clinical student. These tutorials can be an excellent way of consolidating and testing your knowledge.

Each part of the clinical course usually starts with a block of lectures, following which, students are dispersed to attachments at Addenbrooke's Hospital or elsewhere within. Teaching is still very much clinically based, so students get very good exposure to patients.

Assessment

On the preclinical course, you sit exams in May/June at the end of Part IA and Part IB. Each subject has a multiple choice/short answer paper and a practical paper (which count both towards your BA and your 2nd MB) and an essay paper (which counts only towards your BA). You need to pass the 2nd MB in each subject to be able to enter clinical school, and need an honours class in Part IA, Part IB, and your chosen Part II for an honours BA. Although your final BA class depends only upon your Part II results, your Part IA and Part IB results obviously affect how easily you get onto your chosen clinical course. Graduate course students only sit the 2nd MB papers.

All future intakes to the clinical school will sit the new final MB, to be introduced in 2005. This will cover medicine, surgery, and obstetrics and gynaecology, and will involve a multiple choice paper, an extended matching paper, a short answer paper and two OSCEs (objective structured clinical examinations), one on clinical skills and one on communication skills. Final MB pathology will still form a separate exam taken earlier in the course. There are also assessments at the end of each clinical attachment, which have to be passed before sitting finals.

Intercalated degrees

As completing the BA is compulsory, all non-graduate-entry preclinical students intercalate. It is a requirement for the BA to be resident in Cambridge, so you cannot intercalate elsewhere. An exception to this is a Cambridge–MIT (Massachusetts Institute of Technology) exchange scheme, taking 3 medical students each year, who then stay at Cambridge for their clinical studies.

Eight or nine clinical students each year follow the MB PhD programme, for which they apply after being accepted into clinical school but before starting the course.

Special study modules and electives

On both the standard clinical and graduate courses there is a 7-week elective period: 95% of students go abroad. Limited funding (£80–£200) is available for electives from the clinical school, although students have to compete for these, and there may also be some assistance from your college.

Neither the preclinical nor the clinical course currently has special study modules, although there is a limited choice of options for the last few weeks of Part IB. The graduate course has introduced special study modules; however, so far they are all compulsory blocks of the course.

Erasmus

An Erasmus exchange is not normally possible during the preclinical course due to the requirement to be resident in Cambridge, and does not form part of the clinical course. Currently the only overseas travel opportunity apart from the elective is the MIT exchange scheme mentioned above.

Facilities

Library   Cambridge is not short of libraries. The Medical Library is a part of the University Library, based at the Clinical School, and has multiple copies of many undergraduate clinical textbooks, as well as specialist books. The University Library is a copyright library, so officially should get a copy of every book published in Britain, of which all the medical books should end up in the Medical Library. Clinical students can borrow books for up to 4 weeks at a time. In addition, each college has a library, usually well stocked with preclinical textbooks in particular, and each department has a library. Some of the college or departmental libraries have 24-hour access; the Medical Library is open from 8 am to 10 pm on weekdays.

Computers   There are computers everywhere in Cambridge and all students have an email account and access to the central computing facilities. The colleges also have computing networks available to their students, and many departments also have facilities available to their Part II students. Most college rooms have a network access point, and at least one college provides a computer (not necessarily the most up-to-date model!) for all its students living in. The Clinical School has computers specifically for clinical students as well as others for use by anyone, and a wireless area network for those with suitably equipped laptops or palmtops. There is also a set of terminals spread around Addenbrooke's Hospital set up for students to access teaching resources while on the wards.

Welfare

Student support

All students have to be members of a college, and their college will allocate them to a tutor and a director of studies. The tutor's academic subject may be unrelated to medicine, and they may be responsible for students from a wide range of courses. Their duties cover welfare matters such as finance and housing, and general pastoral care. The Director of Studies in Preclinical Medicine may be medically qualified or may be a scientist in one of the preclinical disciplines, and is responsible for students' academic progress and arranging supervisors in the various preclinical subjects. Directors of studies in clinical medicine are normally medically qualified and are supposed to provide academic advice and support, plus advice on matters such as elective placements.

During the preclinical course there is a strong emphasis on the college as a focus for academic issues, although it is always possible to contact the various lecturers or course organisers for each subject. There is also a Director of Medical and Veterinary Education who oversees the preclinical course. During the clinical course the focus shifts to the Clinical School, and the Director of Medical Education in the Clinical School is normally a student's first point of contact over an academic issue.

Most colleges also have chaplains who are available for the pastoral support of students from any background. There are numerous university-linked organisations involved in student support, including the University Counselling Service, CUSU (Cambridge University Students' Union), and various student run organisations.

Accommodation

Quality and cost vary with the college (and the wealth of the college), but it is often difficult to find out the position before you apply – it comes to be a "small print" issue in most of the colleges' entries in the university prospectus. Most undergraduates can expect to live in college for at least 2 out of the 3 preclinical years, and have college-provided accommodation, often in college-owned houses around Cambridge, for the other year. One hangover from the past is that most colleges continue to provide staff, known as "bedders", to clean student rooms – having to do your own cleaning if you move into privately-owned accommodation can be a shock! The standard at its worst is definitely bearable. At its best you are unlikely to get better rooms anywhere else, and it is probably better than your own room at home!

Many colleges will also provide accommodation, albeit usually not in college, for the clinical years, and students coming from preclinical courses elsewhere to join the clinical course can expect to have something provided for year 1 at least. Many clinical students who have already been at Cambridge for the preclinical years decide to rent a shared house in the private sector at this point, and many houses get handed on from one group of clinical students to another. This tends to cost between £50 and £60 per week for a middle-of-the-range house, usually shared by three or four people.

Placements

The preclinical lectures and practicals for Parts IA and IB are held on the science sites in the centre of Cambridge, and are within walking distance of most of the central colleges. Supervisions take place in your own college or in your supervisor's department.

All the teaching on the clinical course is based at Addenbrooke's Hospital, which is situated 2.5 miles south-east of the city centre. Many students live close to Addenbrooke's and walk in; however, it can easily be reached by bus or bicycle from anywhere in Cambridge. Parking on the hospital site can be a nightmare.

On the standard clinical course there are regional attachments in up to a maximum of 6 out of the 11 Phase I and II placements. In Phase III, half of the time is spent at Addenbrooke's and half in a district general hospital. Accommodation at these placements is provided. Students are usually allocated attachments; however, if a student is heavily involved in a university sport, they can arrange to remain in Addenbrooke's for the majority of firms.

Location of clinical placement/name of hospital	Distance away from medical school (miles)	Difficulty getting there on public transport*	Accommodation available
Hinchingbrooke Hospital, Huntingdon	26	+	Yes
Ipswich Hospital	58	++	Yes
James Paget Hospital, Great Yarmouth	87	++	Yes
Milton Keynes Hospital	48	++	Yes
Papworth Hospital	14	+	Yes

*Ease of accessibility: +, set your alarm clock early; ++, long journey

Sports and social 🏆

City life

With its undeniable beauty and rich history, Cambridge is an inspiring city to work and live in. Undergraduates during term time, graduates and tourists at all times, and, of course, the local residents provide an ever-changing and colourful population superimposed on secluded college cloisters, colonies of student houses, and a busy town centre. On a more practical note, all the usual student needs are provided for within a 15-minute cycle ride or less. Take your pick from the central market, essential supermarkets, and a wide range of chain stores, the excellent Arts Theatre, Corn Exchange and Guildhall, as well as a number of cinemas – college, arthouse, and mainstream. The river soon meanders to open countryside in either direction and, finally, many routes lead out of Cambridge to London (and its attractions) as well as the rest of the country.

Cambridge is not without the dangers of violence and crime and, like most places, these problems are often associated with last orders on a Friday or Saturday night. However, there are no notorious districts and students' property insurance premiums confirm Cambridge as one of the safest places to live and study.

University life

Cambridge life is a heady mix in terms of inhabitants and surroundings. The collegiate system means that in the preclinical years you get to meet students doing a wide variety of subjects, and not just medics. Although the course does place a workload on you, there is time to do plenty of other things, such as sport – in particular rowing – and music, which are well represented throughout the university. There is much more of a "medical school" feel to the clinical stage, with most students living nearer the hospital and away from their colleges. The small year group sizes mean that by the end of the course everyone gets to know one another.

Entertainment is provided at a variety of levels, and may be society-, college-, clinical school-, or university-based. If that is not enough, then there are many shows and concerts put on by non-university establishments in the town. Cambridge is very different from other universities in that there is no central Student Union bar where everyone accumulates. There are bars in each college and student nights during the week at the various Cambridge hot spots. Formal hall meals are a prominent feature of the Cambridge social scene. This is a three-course meal in a college dining hall costing between £3 and £9. Students wear gowns, Latin is muttered, and a gong sounds. It is hard to believe that this becomes normality, but it's great fun and brilliant to keep tradition alive; it's just a nightmare when it's 5 minutes before graduation and you find 3-year-old food ingrained in your gown!

The MedSoc is the fourth largest student society and works to make sure preclinical medics have a good time. Every year there is a Christmas dinner, and other activities such as "bops", barbecues, and pub crawls are also organised. In addition, each college usually has its own medical society which hosts a number of dinners each year and provides ample opportunity to socialise on a less academic level with college fellows. The clinical students' society arranges social events for clinical students, often sponsored by insurance societies hoping to get you to stay signed up with them post qualification. On top of this, there is a whole host of opportunities to be involved in other societies, from drama (the famous Cambridge Footlights) and music to karate and gliding – so the chances are you can find something you will enjoy doing.

Sports life

Almost every sport is catered for at the university level. Facilities at college level vary, but at best include huge playing fields, a multi-gym, and squash courts. Boat clubs, football, rugby, and cricket tend to have the largest shares of the college budgets. Also, it does not matter how good or bad you are, there is always an opportunity to take part in whatever you choose. During the preclinical stage sport is college-based and there is fierce intercollegiate rivalry. The clinical school has a sports society (known as "The Sharks") and there is a sport and fitness centre situated on the hospital site to which all students are given free membership.

Finally, another popular sport in Cambridge is punting. Whether you like to get physical or simply recline, enjoy the cool breeze and listen to punt chauffeurs telling elaborate lies to awe-struck tourists, you will love punting!

Fascinating fact: The teaching of medicine at Cambridge dates back to 1540 when Henry VIII endowed the university's first Professorship of Physics. However, it took another 436 years until the School of Clinical Medicine opened in 1976.

Great things about Cambridge 👍

- The collegiate system means that you get to meet students doing a wide variety of subjects.
- The supervision system ensures that you are able to get help with any academic difficulties, helps to make sure that you are able to keep up with the course, and gives

you substantially more individual tuition than most medical schools. It also makes sure you do the work!
- The social life in Cambridge is brilliant. Every society and college hosts dinners and events, and there is always something to do.
- May week! Actually in June, after the preclinical exams. A week of celebrating, winding down, and college balls! After all this, you have 3 months (in the preclinical years) to skip off into the sunset completely free of work worries.
- The cost of living is relatively low, especially for those in college accommodation, and the proximity of all the necessary amenities makes Cambridge an ideal place to spend life as a student. Additionally, there are many funds/bursaries available to all students for travel, study, and extracurricular activities.

Bad things about Cambridge

- Cambridge is highly academic and can appear a very competitive learning environment, especially just prior to exams, which for some students can be rather stressful. It is common to have 5 hours to complete three essays, a rowing outing in 10 minutes, and a thumping head from the previous night's antics. This is known as "fifth week blues" and affects most students.
- Living in college can be frustrating, as the rules and regulations that the college enforces can make some individuals feel as though they are not being treated like an adult. However, this is a trade-off for having cheap accommodation without the hassle of deposits, landlords, and paying utility bills.
- The course is intensive and it can be easy to fall behind. Although the preclinical terms are short (only 8 weeks of study), they can be very tiring, but this is made up for by longer holidays.
- If you wish to meet patients as soon as you start studying medicine, you will have to wait 3 years. However, if you wish to get the "science" sorted out before you start clinical medicine, the course will suit you.
- The tourists – though admittedly they do generate a lot of income for the town and the colleges – tend to get under your skin and manage to appear almost anywhere and at any time (including occasionally in lectures!).

Further information

Cambridge Admissions Office (CAO)
Kellet Lodge
Tennis Court Road
Cambridge CB2 1QJ
Tel: 01223 333308
Fax: 01223 366383
Email: admissions@cam.ac.uk
Web: http://www.cam.ac.uk/CambUniv/undergrad/

University of Cambridge School of Clinical Medicine
Box 111
Addenbrooke's Hospital
Hills Road
Cambridge CB2 2SP
Tel: 01223 336700
Fax: 01223 336709
Email: school-enquiries@medschl.cam.ac.uk
Web: http://www.medschl.cam.ac.uk./pages/admission.html

Graduate course information
Contact via one of the participating colleges:
Admissions Officer
Hughes Hall
Cambridge CB1 2EW
Tel: 01223 334 897
Fax: 01223 311 179
Email: ugadmissions@hughes.cam.ac.uk
Web: http://www.hughes.cam.ac.uk/admissions/ugradadmit.html

Admissions Officer
Lucy Cavendish College (women only)
Cambridge CB3 0BU
Tel: 01223 330 280
Fax: 01223 332 178
Email: lcc-admission@lists.cam.ac.uk
Web: http://www.lucy-cav.cam.ac.uk/
http://www.lucy-cav.cam.ac.uk/Admissions/Postgraduate/Grad_medical_course.html

The Undergraduate Admissions Tutor
Wolfson College
Barton Road
Cambridge CB3 9BB
Tel: 01223 335 900
Fax: 01223 335 908
Email: ug-admissions@wolfson.cam.ac.uk
Web: http://www.wolfson.cam.ac.uk/

http://www.wsufftrust.org.uk/CGC/default.asp
http://www.cam.ac.uk/cambuniv/ugprospectus/courses/medicine5.html

Additional application information

Average A-level requirements	• AAA in science/maths
Average Scottish Higher requirements	• Check with individual colleges admissions tutors
Graduate entry requirements	• 2:1 in any discipline
Make-up of interview panel	• Each college varies. Usually involves tutorial, science/clinical staff
Months in which interviews are held	• December
Proportion of overseas students	• 7%
Proportion of mature students	• 5%
Proportion of graduate students	• Information unavailable
Faculty's view of students taking a gap year	• Acceptable if used constructively
Proportion of students taking intercalated degrees	• All students study for three preclinical years, including BA Hons
Possibility of direct entrance to clinical phase	• All students are interviewed again before entry to the clinical school. About 10% of the clinical school's intake is from other UK medical schools
Fees for overseas students	• £10 596 pa (preclinical) £19 614 pa (clinical) plus £2000–£3000 (college fees)
Fees for graduates	• See Chapter 6
Ability to transfer to other medical schools	• Standard course: transfer common between preclinical and clinical courses. Graduate course: transfer not possible
Assistance for elective funding	• Small bursaries available
Assistance for travel to attachments	• LEA-funded students: normally one return trip/attachment outside Cambridge paid for
Access and hardship funds	• Administered centrally, no funds set aside for medical students in particular
Weekly rent	• £55
Pint of lager	• £1.50
Cinema	• £4.50
Nightclub	• Free–£15

Cardiff University Medical School (merging in August 2004 with University of Wales College of Medicine)

Key facts	Cardiff		Swansea
	Premedical	Undergraduate	Graduate
Course length	6 years	5 years	4 years
Total number of medical undergraduates	14	1335	70 in 2005
Applicants in 2003	191	1459	450
Interviews given in 2003	30	c 800	To be decided
Places available in 2003	14	298	35
Places available in 2004	14	298	70
Open days 2004	21 April (annual open day) February/June/July/September/ November (medical school visits)		28 April
Entrance requirements	ABB (370 points)	ABB (370 points)	Preferably 2:1 in any discipline
Mandatory subjects	Two GCSE sciences	Two science A-levels with chemistry or biology	None
Male:female ratio	31:69	33:67	New course
Is an exam included in the selection process? If yes, what form does this exam take?	No	No	Yes, GAMSAT
Qualification gained	MBBCh		

103

The University of Wales College of Medicine (UWCM) in Cardiff is a member college of the University of Wales responsible for the provision of teaching of medicine, dentistry, nursing, radiography, physiotherapy, occupational therapy, and other professions allied to medicine. This provides a unique opportunity for interprofessional health education, plus a Students' Union solely for these students. Increasing links and an imminent merger with Cardiff University will increase yet further the facilities available to medical students. The university has strong links with all hospitals in Wales, offering clinical placements across the principality. Students from all walks of life – mature, overseas, Welsh, and non-Welsh – make a varied student body, providing a peer group for almost any person. The university is ideally located for the leisure/ recreation/social facilities available in this small, yet friendly capital city.

Education

The course has been following the new curriculum since October 1995. The new course is guided by five themes and delivered through 11 subject panels, with practical experience gained through clinical modules. Year 1 is the foundation year, introducing basic clinical and scientific skills and knowledge, with years 2 and 3 developing them further. Years 4 and 5 place a greater emphasis on clinical experience in preparing for the role of house officer. Teaching is provided through core and special study module components.

A graduate course, based in Swansea for the first 2 years will be introduced in September 2004. These two years will consist of systems-based learning of the basic clinical sciences at the university, and basic clinical skills on the wards. In years 3 and 4, the students will join the cohorts of 4th and 5th years from the Cardiff-based course and do clinical attachments across Wales.

Teaching

A combination of lectures, tutorials, small group sessions, and self-directed learning makes up the bulk of the learning. Anatomy is learnt by hands-on human dissection and taught using demonstrated dissection and prosections. Various computer-assisted learning programs are used, mainly as a revision medium and for tutorial support. Firm sizes vary depending on the hospital: five to six in the main teaching hospitals, and usually two in the district general hospitals (DGHs) (varying from one to four).

Assessment

Examinations take place at the end of years 1, 3, 4, and 5, with resits being available in the years 1 and 3. Continuous assessment and the satisfactory completion of all coursework and special study modules are a feature of the examination process.

Intercalated degrees

Intercalated degrees are available to one-third of the year, and can be done after years 2, 3, and 4. There is a choice of subjects, including basic medical sciences (anatomy, physiology, biochemistry), or more clinically orientated modular degrees in medical sciences.

Special study modules and electives

Special study modules make up 24–30% of the timetable throughout the 5 years. An 8-week period of elective study, either in the UK or abroad, is undertaken in the final year as part of the normal block rotation. Students pursue an original research project on any subject of personal interest and provide a written report of their elective experience.

Erasmus

The College participates in the SOCRATES ERASMUS (European Community Action Scheme for the Mobility of University Students) exchange programme funded by the European Union. Opportunities exist for students to study for 3 months in France, Germany, Finland, Holland, Italy, Sweden, and Romania.

Facilities

Library   The library facilities in the main teaching hospital consist of three separate libraries, two 24-hour reading rooms and a 40-PC 24-hour computer room. The availability of texts and journals is excellent. Students also have access to the library and computing facilities of the University of Wales, Cardiff University, and many other libraries in most hospitals.

Computers   There are adequate computer facilities on site, and in most outlying hospitals. Some tuition is given initially, and all submitted work is expected to be word processed.

Clinical skills   Cardiff has a new skills laboratory which is heavily used. It is a key focus for the new curriculum.

Welfare

Student support

UWCM is very student friendly and actively encourages and acts upon the views of its students. Monthly meetings between year reps and the Dean occur where students' grievances are voiced in an informal setting. Students are also represented on all the curriculum planning committees. Being part of the University of Wales allows students access to its general counselling and welfare services, as well as pastoral care within the faculty.

Accommodation

Accommodation is provided in year 1 by Cardiff University. There is space for all first-years in halls. The standards are high, with over 50% of accommodation being less than 5 years old, and two-thirds are en suite. There is ample good-quality private housing for rent, with prices ranging from £45 to £55 a week. Cardiff Council runs a house renting registration scheme, which aims to monitor and license rented accommodation in the city.

Location of clinical placement/name of hospital	Distance away from medical school (miles)	Difficulty getting there on public transport*	Accommodation available
University Hospital of Wales, Cardiff	0	+	No
Royal Glamorgan Hospital, Llantrisant	12	++	No
Princess of Wales Hospital, Bridgend	20	++	Yes
Singleton Hospital, Swansea	40	+++	Yes
Ysbyty Gwynedd, Bangor	260	+++	Yes

*Ease of accessibility: +, set your alarm clock early; ++, long journey; +++, car is a must

Placements

The medical school is based on two sites approximately 1.5 miles apart: the Cardiff School of Biosciences (part of Cardiff University) and UWCM at the University Hospital of Wales. Community-based teaching in practices in and around Cardiff forms a substantial part of the course. Hospitals throughout Wales are used for teaching, ensuring an excellent student–patient ratio. It also provides an opportunity for students to see all of the different parts of Wales, and gain more of an idea where to apply for jobs a few years down the line. Bangor is the most distant of the DGHs used, being 260 miles away from Cardiff. Attachments in general practice include some time spent at a rural practice somewhere in Wales. Travel subsidies are available from the college, and accommodation is provided in all DGHs outside Cardiff.

Sports and social 🏆

City life

Cardiff is a very student-friendly city. UWCM, Cardiff University, UW Institute Cardiff, and the Welsh College of Music and Drama combine to make a student population of over 26 000. Most clubs/pubs/theatres, etc host student nights with special rates for NUS card holders. The city also has plenty of parks and open spaces, so there is always somewhere to relax and sunbathe, especially in the summer. As the capital, Cardiff has all the attractions that you would expect of a large city while being small enough to make you feel at home. The local countryside is very beautiful, and all outdoor activities are available. The development of Cardiff Bay and the Welsh Assembly has given added excitement to the atmosphere in the city.

University life

Medical students are members of their own Students' Club, which provides sporting facilities/teams, its own fleet of minibuses, and its own bar, where drinks are often the cheapest in Cardiff! The Students' Club organises one staff/student dinner a year, six balls, and many other social events, ranging from top-name bands, comedians, long-distance pub crawls, and tours around the UK – all attended by a mix of medics, dentists, nurses, radiographers, and physiotherapy students. A wide range of clubs and societies are available, including climbing, orchestra, canoeing, and martial arts. There are also religious groups such as the Islamic Society and the Christian Medical Fellowship. Each year the students organise a charity revue called "Anaphylaxis" and publish *Medrag* to raise money for local charities. In 1992 the Students' Union started its own charity, BACCUP. Each year a limited number of UWCM students have the opportunity to travel out to Belarus to work in an orphanage for children with special needs. Students also have access to the much greater facilities provided by Cardiff University and its Students' Union.

Student life can be very hectic, juggling work commitments with the variety of sports and clubs offered by UWCM Students' Club. The majority of teams, clubs, and societies are fully funded by the Club, including the provision of five minibuses for the use of its members. "Medclub", UWCM's own bar/club, provides a friendly, social, and cheap venue for the post-match celebrations, and a very cheap source of alcohol for those not partaking in the sporting scene! It is also the venue for some of the craziest scenes you're likely to find during freshers' week. There is also the impressive Cardiff Students' Union, with its two bars, 1800 capacity nightclub, live music venue, and snooker/pool hall. As a capital city, Cardiff offers excellent sport, leisure, and recreational facilities. The Millennium Stadium hosts the FA Cup and the Worthington Cup Finals, the Six Nations rugby matches, as well as a number of live music gigs. Cardiff also has a great range of shops, pubs, clubs, and a redeveloped seafront at Cardiff Bay. Living in Cardiff allows easy access to beautiful and varied scenery, including the Brecon Beacons National Park.

Sports life

The Club has a large number of teams, some of which gain great success far beyond that expected of a small university. Our rugby team has won the MedSchools Cup many times! Most teams compete in the various BUSA interuniversity competitions, intermedical school competitions, and some local leagues. The Students' Club has a multigym, pool, and snooker tables. Besides the facilities on offer by the dedicated Students' Union of UWCM, students have the benefit of using the sports and Union facilities of Cardiff University.

Fascinating fact: The Daddy of evidence-based medicine and randomised controlled trials, Archie Cochrane, pioneered epidemiology as a science while working for the Welsh National School of Medicine (now UWCM) here in Cardiff.

Great things about Cardiff

- Students are members of the Students' Unions at UWC (Cardiff University) and UWCM, allowing access to both Med Club and the bars and nightclub at Cardiff University. This allows medical students to socialise with non-medics as well as medics.
- A lot of interactions (socially and academically!) between students of all years, and with dental, nursing, physio students, etc.
- All the advantages of living in an expanding and vibrant capital city without the usual costs.
- Using all Welsh hospitals keeps firm sizes low and student/patient ratios high.
- An excellent course with a great balance between problem-based learning, lectures, and clinical experience.

Bad things about Cardiff

- The large year group size means it can be difficult to get to know all fellow students individually.
- The wait for coursework to be returned is often long.
- Distances between hospitals and the accessibility of some rural hospitals make travelling very awkward and time consuming, unless you have a car.
- Clinical placements in years 4 and 5 can make it hard to see your non-medic friends (and medic friends not with you on placement) regularly.
- The weather!

Further information

Undergraduate Admissions Officer
University of Wales College of Medicine
Heath Park
Cardiff CF4 4XN
Tel: 029 2074 2027
Fax. 029 2074 2914
Email: uwcmadmissions@cf.ac.uk
Web: http://www.uwcm.ac.uk
Open days: February, April, June, July

Swansea Clinical School
Grove Building
University of Wales Swansea
Singleton Park
Swansea
SA2 8PP
Tel: 01792 513 400
Fax: 01792 513 430
Email: p.g.maull@swan.ac.uk
Web: www.medicine.swan.ac.uk

Additional application information

Average A-level requirements	• Two science A-levels (chemistry, biology, physics, maths, statistics) at AB grades, one of which must be chemistry or biology. Non-science subject encouraged excluding general studies
Average Scottish Higher requirements	• AAAAB including English language, chemistry, physics and biology. Two Advanced Highers at AA including chemistry
Graduate entry requirements	• 2:1 in any discipline, 2:2 considered when applicant also has a higher degree
Make-up of interview panel	• Mix of hospital specialist, GP, scientist, health professional, lay person, student
Months in which interviews are held	• November–March (undergraduate course) December–April (graduate course)
Proportion of overseas students	• 7%
Proportion of mature students	• 11%
Proportion of graduate students	• 8%
Faculty's view of students taking a gap year	• Welcomed
Proportion of students taking intercalated degrees	• 20%
Possibility of direct entrance to clinical phase	• No
Fees for overseas students	• £18 350
Fees for graduates	• See Chapter 6
Ability to transfer to other medical schools	• Applications considered in their own right. Financial and family health reasons are usually accepted. However, transfers require a mutual acceptance from the receiving medical school
Assistance for elective funding	• Several bursaries available to compete for
Assistance for travel to attachments	• Free transport provided to placements in year 3, clinical placement costs reimbursed in years 4 and 5. A car-sharing scheme is in the pipeline!
Access and hardship funds	• Financial contingency funds available to those in serious financial difficulty
Weekly rent	• £50–60
Pint of lager	• £1.50
Cinema	• £5
Nightclub	• £5

Dundee

Key facts	Premedical	Undergraduate
Course length	6 years	5 years
Total number of medical undergraduates	5	807
Applicants in 2003	80	1169
Interviews given in 2003	13	550
Places available in 2003	Up to 10	154
Places available in 2004	Up to 10	154
Open days 2004	23 June	
Entrance requirements	AAB A-levels in non-science subjects, or AAAAB Scottish Highers in non-science subjects	AAB
Mandatory subjects	Non-science	Chemistry
Male:female ratio	–	43:57
Is an exam included in the selection process?	No	No
If yes, what form does this exam take?		
Qualification gained		MBChB

Dundee is a modern, friendly and forward-thinking medical school with an international reputation. Dundee medics are known for being easy going and down-to-earth; intake is approximately 40% Scottish, 40% Irish (Northern Ireland and Republic of Ireland), 10% English, and 10% international. Dundee is extremely supportive of graduate/mature students and encourages applications from a wide variety of backgrounds. Indeed graduate and mature students make up over 16% of every year, and each year also has about seven entrants from the premedical course. The new curriculum was introduced in 1993 and enables good staff–student interaction with achievable learning goals and a realistic workload. Clinical teaching begins in year 2. Many aspects of the course at Dundee have received plaudits from the Scottish Higher Education Funding Council and the biomedical research programme is world renowned. Ninewells Hospital, the largest purpose-built teaching hospital in Europe, is built on a green park campus on the banks of the River Tay.

Education 📖

The first cohort from the new-style course graduated in 2000 and the integrated course is well established. Teaching is structured around body systems. Year 1 (Phase I) covers normal body structure and function and is taught at the main campus. First-year students also visit patients in the community and do a basic emergency care course which includes training in cardiopulmonary resuscitation. During year 1, students are divided into groups for tutorials and practicals. Groups then change in year 2 for the Practising Medicine (clinical) programme, which helps students get to know more members of their year. Phase II (years 2 and 3) and III (years 4 and 5) are based at Ninewells Hospital. Phase II concentrates on abnormal structure and function, and phase III deals with solving the problems of abnormal structure and function. The curriculum requires mastery (a pass grade of 75%) of relevant facts, clinical skills, and the correct attitude. Special study modules are a key component, but are assessed using different criteria.

Teaching

The systems-based course promotes independent learning. Each block comes with a study guide, which includes core material and a summary of the clinical skills to be mastered each week, problem-based questions, tutorial questions, and references. Phase I teaching is a mixture of lectures, dissection, laboratories, behavioural sciences, and tutorials. There is no use of animals or animal tissues in practicals. Phase II includes lectures, clinical skills, ward teaching (about eight students to a ward group), small group work, and primary care medicine. Multidisciplinary teaching takes place between the medical and nursing schools for ethics, and between the medical and midwifery schools for some parts of the Phase II reproduction, growth, and development block.

Phase III is primarily clinical and includes a house officer apprenticeship in year 5. This provides extensive training so that students will be competent house officers, and often takes place in the hospital where the PRHO year will be spent.

Teaching at Dundee has recently been rated excellent by the Scottish Higher Education Funding Council and is well thought of in GMC assessments.

Assessment

Exams consist of written papers comprising constructed response question (CRQ) and extended matching item (EMI) components, an objective structured clinical examination (OSCE) and a portfolio exam. Finals are taken at the end of year 4.

In CRQs students are given a brief patient history followed by some questions about, for example, possible differential diagnoses. After this more information is provided and the examinee is asked to refine their diagnosis and management. This process continues until the student has been led through the patient case. In contrast EMIs consist of approximately six questions and 15 answers, which students then need to match up.

In-course assessment consists of a literature review task running throughout year 1 and a research assignment in year 4.

Intercalated degrees

Intercalated degrees are optional and are taken by invitation from the faculty. Subjects typically include medical and social sciences, but BAs can also be taken. Dundee is the only school to offer a Bachelor of Medical Science (BMSc) in Forensic Medicine and Orthopaedic Technology. A few students take an intercalated degree course elsewhere in the UK, typically at one of the London schools.

Special study modules and electives

Over 42 SSMs are advertised on the medical school website, and you can also design your own. Overseas options are available and staff are very supportive of individually designed SSMs taking place in their clinics or laboratories. Year 5 kicks off with a 7-week elective (10 weeks if the 3-week vacation is included!). It's up to you to organise your own programme. Information and help regarding funding are widely available.

Erasmus

The medical school does not participate in the Erasmus scheme. However, SSMs provide an opportunity to travel abroad and the medical school offer an SSM in France.

Facilities

Library   Recommended texts for first year are housed in a large multifaculty library on the main campus. Books for students in years 2–5 are housed at the Medical Library at Ninewells Hospital. Normal opening hours are Monday to Friday 9 am–10 pm; Saturday and Sunday 9 am–6 pm. There is good availability of reference books, but be prepared to reserve some books in advance. Libraries open later as the academic year progresses.

Computers   There is extensive computer access at both Ninewells (open 8 am–11 pm all week) and the main campus. Facilities include computer-assisted learning (CAL) tutorials, microbiology laboratory summaries, MCQs, MRI/CT/x ray imaging, revision sessions, email and internet. Classes in IT skills are laid on for the nervous!

Clinical skills   The purpose-built clinical skills centre opened in 1997. It provides multiprofessional teaching to small groups in areas such as communication and history taking; professional attitudes and ethics; physical examination and laboratory skills; diagnostics and therapeutics; and resuscitation. The centre is open 9 am–5 pm for teaching and drop-in revision sessions. The clinical and administrative staff are extremely supportive and proactive, and run a book-in service for clinical skills revision sessions. Facilities include access to anatomical models and mannequins; diagnostic, therapeutic and resuscitation equipment; videos; simulated and real patients; and telemedicine links.

Typical clinical skills sessions in Phase II (years 2 and 3) are generally good fun, last 2 hours, and allow students to develop confidence and competence in clinical skills before going on to the wards.

Welfare

Student support

The staff tend to be friendly, approachable, and supportive. They really do make an effort to ensure that students get the extra clinical training, core knowledge, and time for small group work required by the new curriculum. A new staff–student leisure facility at Ninewells was completed in 1998, and a house officer facility was completed in 1996. The School of Nursing and Midwifery joined the Faculty of Medicine and Dentistry in 1997. Each student is assigned a personal and academic tutor. There is a Special Needs Coordinator, based at Student Welfare on the main campus. The Dean is very approachable and student friendly, and operates an open-door policy. Likewise, lecturers and clinicians are approachable, and typically put a lot of work into designing and teaching each block. All medical freshers are sent a student-produced *Student Survival Guide*, which includes information on the course, social and sporting activities, and local transport, etc. The students run a Senior–Junior scheme where students from later years support the students from earlier years. There is also a very active Medical Students' Council, which regularly attends faculty meetings to voice student opinion. The council runs a careers fair, women in medicine evening, annual symposium, electives evening, and PRHO meetings for students. A good indicator of staff–student relations is the number of staff who regularly attend year, club, and hospital balls. The medical school has good wheelchair access.

Accommodation

There are two halls on campus. Belmont is a large 1900s catered hall of residence next to the Union, the sports centre, and the library. Airlie is a smaller self-catering hall on the other side of the Union and the library. Peterson House and Seabraes Flats are a 1-minute stumble from campus. They are both self-catering; the latter was built in 1996, and contains flats with en-suite bathrooms. The West Park Centre is halfway between the town and Ninewells in the leafy west end of Dundee, and offers both catered and self-catering halls. This accommodation was also built in 1996. The catered accommodation consists of self-contained flats with phones, en-suite bathrooms, colour TVs, and computer links to the university internet. Most first-years live in halls. Private accommodation costs around £40–50 per week, generally in the west end of Dundee, and standards are pretty good.

Placements

Year 1 is based at the main campus with occasional visits to Ninewells. Years 2–5 are hospital-based. Ninewells Hospital is about 3 miles from the town and main campus on the Firth of Tay. Wards have spectacular river views. Many students walk (30 minutes), cycle, or drive to the hospital, but numerous buses run right to the front door (fare 95p), and there is now a free university bus running every hour from campus to Ninewells and back. Car parking is available but costs £1.50 per day or around £20 per month by direct debit if you get a key fob.

Location of clinical placement/name of hospital	Distance away from medical school (miles)	Difficulty getting there on public transport*	Accommodation available
Perth	26	+	Yes
Queen Margaret, Dunfermline	50	++	Yes
Airdrie	80	++	Yes
Ayr	110	++	Yes
Whitehaven	300	+++	Yes

*Ease of accessibility: +, set your alarm clock early; ++, long journey; +++, car is a must

In years 2 and 3 ward teaching is at Ninewells Hospital. In years 4 and 5 you get a chance to travel around the UK and see how other hospitals work: up to 5 months of years 4 and 5 can be spent away from Dundee on outblocks if desired. Placements with district general hospitals (DGHs) and GPs are set up around Scotland (including the Highlands and Islands) and the north of England, with free hospital accommodation provided. Guesthouse accommodation or travel expenses are available for many GP placements. A computer matching system allocates students to their peripheral attachments on a best-fit basis, so most students can stay in Dundee if they wish, although for many the experience of peripheral hospital/GP attachments is a highlight.

Sports and social 🏆

City life

Dundee is Scotland's fourth largest city and has a beautiful location on the Firth of Tay. Local sights include the riverside itself; the neighbouring seaside town of Broughty Ferry with its sandy beaches, castle, shops, and pubs; Tentsmuir Forest Park and beaches; Carnoustie; St Andrews (15 miles away); numerous golf courses; and fantastic sunsets. As well as being spectacular, the countryside offers skiing, hill walking, climbing, and numerous water sports. A new shopping centre opened in 2000, vastly improving Dundee's shopping facilities. The city is very student friendly, and the area around the university is very much a student community. Many new small shops, cafés, bars, and clubs have opened on the Perth Road in Dundee's west end over the past 18 months. There is constant building and renovation work in the town. Glasgow, Edinburgh, and Aberdeen are all within reach for a weekend, 1–1.5 hours drive or train journey away.

University life

Dundee University Medical Society (DUMS) sponsors freshers' week events, and puts on many social bashes and trips throughout the year. DUMS tends to form a large part of a medic's social life, especially in the earlier years. Each year also has its own Yearclub to put on events – for example end of year balls, fancy dress parties, nights out, pub golf, and slave auctions – to raise money for charity. Ceilidhs (Scottish dancing) are very popular and are a great ice-breaker. Lessons are given for the uninitiated. Each Yearclub organises a halfway dinner (weekend away at a hotel with ball, etc) guess when – halfway through the course – and their own graduation ball (there is also a university graduation ball). The Students Union building has been refurbished and hosts packed-out club nights through the week, and is very popular with medics. Local pubs abound (some hosting live music) and the beer is cheap. The Dundee Repertory Theatre is active nationally, and hosts plays, musicals, and jazz festivals. The popular Dundee Contemporary Arts Centre (DCA) provides two screens for "arthouse" films, a large art gallery, café and wine bar, all right beside the university. There are also two multiplex cinemas, an Odeon and an UGC. The Duncan of Jordanstone Art School is part of the main campus, adding diversity to the student population, and their summer final-year show is always a sell-out. The university also has the usual wide variety of societies and sporting organisations.

Sports life

The sports centre now boasts the largest university indoor facilities in Scotland. Outdoor pitches are based at the scenic and windy Riverside Drive. The university has a very active and varied sports scene, with a good level of competition at both Scottish and British university level. The medical school has its own teams in football, rugby, and netball. Competitions are organised against other Scottish medical schools. Medics often play for both the medical school and the university, with the medical school teams being a little less competitive in spirit than the university teams.

Fascinating fact: Dundee medical school is the home to Professor Sir Alfred Cushieri, a pioneer of "keyhole' surgery, and Sir James Black, a Nobel prizewinner in medicine whose work led to the discovery of beta-blockers.

Great things about Dundee

- Good teaching on an established new-style course with early patient exposure.
- Good social life based around DUMS, and a friendly bunch of staff and students means that you can always find something to do.
- Dundee is a cheap, safe, and fun place to live.
- The clinical skills centre is excellent.
- Dundee is surrounded by beautiful countryside, with access to skiing, hill walking, watersports, and places such as St Andrews are close-by for daytrips.

Bad things about Dundee

- It can take some time to get used to the local accent!
- Dundee is not a great centre for shopping.
- From year 2 onwards you are based almost exclusively at Ninewells during the day and may feel a little isolated from the other students on campus.

- It does get cold and windy over the winter.
- It can be difficult to park at Ninewells.

Further information

Information Centre
Admissions and Student Recruitment
2 Airlie Place
The University of Dundee
Nethergate
Dundee DD1 4HN
Tel: 01382 344032 (admissions)
Tel: 01382 344160 (prospectus requests)
Tel: 01382 348111 (international)
Fax: 01382 348150
Email: srs@dundee.ac.uk
Web: http://www.dundee.ac.uk

Additional application information

Average A-level requirements	• ABB (chemistry)
Average Scottish Higher requirements	• AAABB (chemistry)
Graduate entry requirements	• 2:2 in any discipline
Make-up of interview panel	• Members of the Faculty of Medicine
Months in which interviews are held	• December–March
Proportion of overseas students	• 7.5%
Proportion of mature students	• 3%
Proportion of graduate students	• 13%
Faculty's view of students taking a gap year	• Acceptable
Proportion of students taking intercalated degrees	• 6%
Possibility of direct entrance to clinical phase	• None
Fees for overseas students	• £9500 (premedical) £11 800 pa (preclinical) £18 800 pa (clinical)
Fees for graduates	• See Chapter 6
Ability to transfer to other medical schools	• Students are free to transfer to other medical schools if another school has a place for them
Assistance for elective funding	• Dependent on Faculty Funds
Assistance for travel to attachments	• No – responsibility of LEA/ELB/SAAS
Access and hardship funds	• University Hardship Fund available
Weekly rent	• £40–£50
Pint of lager	• Union £1.40; pubs £1.50 upwards
Cinema	• £3.50 with matriculation card at Odeon and UGC
Nightclub	• £2.50. Large selection offering all tastes in music/dance and entertainment

East Anglia

Key facts	Undergraduate
Course length	5 years
Total number of medical undergraduates	220 at present
Applicants in 2003	900
Interviews given in 2003	450
Places available in 2003	110
Places available in 2004	130
Open days 2004	July and October
Entrance requirements	AAB or 2:1
Mandatory subjects	Biology
Male:female ratio	40:60
Is an exam included in the selection process? If yes, what form does this exam take?	No
Qualification gained	MBBS

University of East Anglia (UEA) was opened in 2002 as part of the expansion of medical school places in the UK. It offers an innovative five year programme that includes exposure to primary care from the first week of study.

Education

This brand new medical curriculum follows the university motto, "Do Different". Its innovative, and in some respects, controversial structure places patients at the centre of all learning. Clinical exposure takes place right from the start of the course with integrated teaching at university, in general practice, and in hospitals. Communication skills and an understanding of people are paramount to the way this course addresses disease.

Teaching

The medical curriculum follows systems-based units throughout the 5 years, integrating theory, practical skills, and clinical experience from the very start. University-based teaching fills two-thirds of the time, with Problem-Based Learning (PBL) at the core. Students divide into small groups to discuss weekly case scenarios and, with the guidance of a tutor/facilitator, formulate learning objectives for the relevant topics. The aim of the week is then to gather relevant information to "solve" the cases, incorporating all aspects of medicine while maintaining a patient-centred approach. This is supported during the week by lectures and seminars designed to meet relevant objectives and delivered in the main by consultants and specialists. Anatomy is taught through lectures and seminars, using cadavers as illustration. Dissection is not routinely expected from students but those who wish to do so have an opportunity to dissect in the Student Selected Study sessions (see Special Study Modules, below).

During the time predominantly based at university, one day a week is spent in general practice. These "mini-placements" enable a mixture of patient contact and small group teaching, consolidating the week's learning. Such sessions continue to occur throughout all stages of the course and most students agree that this both reinforces and builds on current knowledge in a "real-world" environment.

The other third of teaching time takes place during the block placement in secondary care that accompanies each unit. Students learn through following patients, a variety of clinics, teaching ward rounds and other clinical experiences. There is also a strong emphasis on the multidisciplinary team working together, with time being spent with nurses, therapists, technicians, and other hospital staff.

Both stages are supported with "Blackboard", the medical school's Virtual Learning Environment. In essence, this is a vast online database comprising every lecture note, timetable, and handout you will ever need! It is also used as a file exchange for group work, and for self-assessment with MCQs.

Multidisciplinary practice is very highly regarded at UEA. In conjunction with the School of Nursing and Midwifery and the School of Allied Health Professions, medical students are obliged to take part in combined professional practice exercises. These occur once a week following a similar format to PBL scenarios and are aimed at promoting communication between, and appreciation of, each profession in the Health Service. Whilst all new students will have compulsory sessions, a successful pilot is also being extended into year 2 to see how such teaching can be used for future years.

At the end of year 5, students will shadow the PRHO job in which they will be employed after graduation. Where possible, the school intends this to be with one of their NHS partners in the region. The medical school plans to offer mentoring and postgraduate study throughout the PRHO period.

Assessment

Each unit is assessed with a mini-OSCE, comprising six or so stations. These vary in content to assess communication, clinical skills, and fundamental medical knowledge. Student Selected Study presentations and paper appraisals (see Special Study Modules, below) are also conducted at the end of each unit for the first 3 years.

At the end of each year is an integrative period, where all previous learning is assessed. This takes the form of a large OSCE, and an Advanced Noticed Questions (ANQ) written paper. In an ANQ, students are given a set of problem cases a week in advance so that they are familiar with the problems before the exam. It may include multiple choice questions. A formal reflective appraisal of the year must also be submitted for assessment.

Intercalated degrees

As the course only opened in 2002, there are, as yet, no students undertaking intercalated degrees at UEA. These are planned for the end of year 3 and will result in the completion of a Masters degree (eg MSc).

Special study modules and electives

All UEA students are obliged to take part in Student Selected Studies (SSS). There are two branches to this line of study, which assess a student's ability to gather, appraise, and present information. During each unit, students will study a topic of their choosing, selected from a list of domains (anatomy, biochemistry, epidemiology, ethics, health economics, law, physiology, psychology, sociology) and relevant to the current unit of study. This is then exhibited to clinical tutors and peers during a short presentation with question and answers. In later years, students will be expected to study an area of interest outside medicine.

The second aspect of SSS runs concurrently with the university-based teaching. A series of lectures and support seminars equips students with the skills and knowledge required to appraise research papers. This is assessed through a formal written appraisal every unit during years 1–3. There are also plans for later years whereby students will design and then conduct a research project for themselves.

An 8-week elective is planned for the end of year 4, with students free to choose the location and nature of clinical experience.

Facilities

The majority of teaching takes place in a purpose-built school on the UEA campus. This attractive centre is brand new, although unfortunately a little on the small side. This leads to overcrowding, especially when more than one year group try to converge between lectures. There is also extensive use of cutting-edge facilities at the Norfolk and Norwich University Hospital (NNUH), which has recently been relocated to modern, custom-built premises just a few minutes walk from campus. Most students are impressed with this exciting facility.

In addition, teaching takes place at the James Paget Hospital in Gorleston and in GP surgeries across the region. The psychiatry module in year 5 will be taught in conjunction with Norfolk Mental Health Trust at their facilities across the county.

Library   The UEA boasts a large library, suitably stocked with copies of all books on the reading list. Students also have access to the hospital libraries at both teaching hospitals, which have a good collection of books on the entire range of medical specialities.

Computers   With widespread use of the Virtual Learning Environment, computer access is inevitably important to all students. The MED building on campus has a 24-hour access computer facility purely for the use of medical students although this can get a little busy, especially during lunchtimes. There is an additional, networked facility at the NNUH exclusively for students on placement, with both rooms having 20 or so terminals. Students are also free to make use of the other campus facilities in the computer centre and the library. Network access is available in all campus residences.

Clinical skills   As part of the Joint Venture programme, the school works very closely with the Norfolk and Norwich University Hospital. This has a designated "ward", set aside for student teaching, which includes a well-equipped clinical skills lab with a variety of equipment. The James Paget Hospital, where some secondary care attachments occur, also has an excellent skills lab with dedicated technicians able and willing to assist.

There is a structured clinical skills programme extending across the 5 years, with gradual addition to the student "armoury" each unit. These begin with basic observation skills and CPR, and progress during relevant units (for example, venepuncture during the haematology unit in year 2). It is hoped that students will complete Advanced Life Support training at the end of year 5.

Communication skills are taught extensively in year 1, with supplementary training periodically thereafter, to add to and refresh students' proficiency.

Welfare

Student support

All the staff at the university, both academic and administrative, are very friendly and approachable, with everyone treated as an equal. That said, each student is assigned a personal adviser from the academic or clinical staff with whom they can discuss personal or academic issues. In addition, there is a student-run mentor scheme similar to that at other universities, whereby medical students in senior years are allocated to new arrivals. It is hoped to extend this across the entire period of study, to create a student "family". Students are also on hand on the days that freshers move in to their accommodation to provide support, advice or a friendly face in the bar.

The School of Medicine, Health Policy and Practice also makes use of the welfare services already provided by the UEA. The Dean of Students is responsible for welfare for the university but extensive services are provided by the Union of UEA Students, including an advice centre and confidential help-line out of hours. Problems for those living on campus can be addressed by Resident Tutors – senior students living in the halls to protect the welfare of residents.

Accommodation

The UEA has arguably one of the most attractive campuses in the country (you can even learn to love the original grey, concrete buildings!). There are trees aplenty, and copious open space for recreation or sunbathing. A large lake ("The UEA Broad") makes for a great revision environment on a sunny day. Residential accommodation on this attractive campus is guaranteed to first-year students, with a range of prices and facilities. On the one hand, the en-suite residences have won architectural awards for brilliance; the other is described as the "Swedish prison". The plush surroundings of the more expensive residences are certainly pleasant to live in, but many students who choose more communal living comment on the excellent camaraderie of their halls. All facilities on campus are self-catering but there are a variety of places to eat.

Norwich is well equipped to deal with student housing and there is a good provision of privately rented houses, flats, and bed-sits. Most of these are in the "Golden Triangle" area about 30 minutes

Location of clinical placement/name of hospital	Distance away from medical school (miles)	Difficulty getting there on public transport*	Accommodation available
Norfolk and Norwich University Hospital	1	+	No
James Paget Hospital	32	+++	No
General Practice attachments	Across Norfolk and Suffolk	+++	No

*Ease of accessibility: +, set your alarm clock early; ++, long journey; +++, car is a must

walk from campus, which has a high student population. New estates are being built in Bowthorpe, also about 30 minutes out, where many students choose to buy houses. There may be limited provision of hospital accommodation, but this is a little on the pricey side.

Placements

Clinical placements begin from the first term and continue right through the 5 years. For two-thirds of each unit, a day a week will be spent in one of the many GP practices across Norfolk and Suffolk. The school provides all transport, although many find the journeys can be long and arduous at times. On the plus side, most students find this day to be the highlight of the week.

Each unit also has one-third teaching in a local hospital. This will usually be the Norfolk and Norwich University Hospital, a new hospital complex a few minutes' walk from campus, or the James Paget Hospital, the local DGH for south Norfolk and north Suffolk. The "Paget" is a far smaller hospital, but welcoming, and many students prefer the quieter, more personal environment. It does, unfortunately, mean a 40-minute coach journey twice a day for the duration of the placement, but again this is provided by the school.

Sports and social 🏆

City life

"Norwich, a Fine City" is how most people are greeted when arriving in the capital of Norfolk. It is large enough to be vibrant and exciting, yet small enough to still reflect its very rural surroundings.

Whilst still a bustling city, Norwich has managed to retain a relaxed and friendly atmosphere. It was once the second largest city in Britain and still proudly displays the castle and most of its other historic remnants in its medieval centre, including two magnificent cathedrals. In sharp contrast, Norwich continues to move forward with the recent opening of The Forum, which holds a library, restaurants, and the local BBC services and looks out over one of the largest open-air markets in the country.

Norwich's surroundings are some of the most attractive and unique anywhere in the world. From the waterways of the Norfolk Broads (a National Park) to the vast expanses of the North Norfolk coastline, this is certainly a region worth exploring. With rail links to London, Cambridge, and the Midlands, many students find it an irresistible environment to live in after graduation.

Norwich's club land becomes the centre of nightlife for East Anglia, although students used to the big city life often complain that it is still "a bit quiet". That said, Norwich's pub/club scene offers a whole range of student nights and low prices.

Shopping is another attraction of this fine city. The large open-air market complements the facilities of the city centre shops in addition to the Castle Mall shopping centre. Holding over 70 shops The Mall is unlikely to impress die-hard shopping fanatics but is certainly one of the largest retail centres in the region, with a good mix of high street chains and local "gems" worth exploring.

University life

The UEA campus is well equipped to provide an almost self-contained environment for those who do not wish to venture from the university. Shops, a post office and of course, the bar, all provide a pleasant, relaxed atmosphere in which to live. There is free student access to the Sainsbury Centre for Visual Arts, the UEA's very own gallery and exhibition centre, for the more culturally inclined.

Last year, the student bar underwent a refit, providing a relaxed, pub-like section but also a contemporary, trendy bar hosting the occasional DJ. Major sports fixtures are displayed on a huge screen at one end of the bar. The atmosphere is generally relaxed and the alcohol is cheap – ideal for a quiet night out, or for some drinking before heading upstairs to the LCR! This is the centre of entertainment at UEA, serving as discotheque, live music venue, comedy hall and "mosh pit". The "Ents" (short for entertainment) team works very hard to ensure that there are always things to do here, and on most weeks, there is some sort of entertainment on offer every night. Some of the biggest names in UK and international music have played at UEA (Coldplay, Mis-teeq, The Darkness, Toploader, Kosheen, The Levellers, Beth Orton, Beverley Knight ... the list goes on!).

There are also plenty of opportunities to get involved away from the bar, and with over 100 clubs and societies to join; there is something on offer for everyone. In addition to the rest of the university, the medical school is already finding *its* voice. With extracurricular activities such as Medical Humanities, MedSIN, and a dedicated MedSoc, the school is definitely making a name for itself within the UEA.

Sports life

UEA as a university is very into its sports. From korfball to lacrosse, there is something to suit most sports fans. In addition, the university runs its own interschool competition called the Ziggurat Challenge. This is a series of events for all abilities and enthusiasms, from die-hard fanatics, to those who would rather just stroll around the campus lake. Unfortunately, medical sports teams are somewhat limited owing to a lack of numbers, although the ultra-keen sports reps have great plans for the future. Presently, medical students also use their sporting energy against staff from the faculty and hospital.

East Anglia

123

UEA boasts 40 acres of dedicated sports field in addition to Astroturf, brand new tennis courts, and local access to water sports. Other facilities include an Olympic-sized swimming pool, indoor arena, gym, climbing wall, National Standard athletics track and so on … all at reduced student rates (£1.25 for gym or swim).

Fascinating fact: Professor Anne Barrett, the President of the Royal College of Oncologists, was the first woman to receive a fellowship from the college. She is a lecturer at the UEA medical school.

Great things about UEA

- Patient contact and consultant-led teaching takes place right from the start of the course, making everything far more relevant and interesting than a text book alone.
- A friendly, warm environment at both school and university level makes UEA great fun for work and play.
- Innovation and participation are encouraged – there is always something exciting to be involved with.
- UEA has fantastic sporting facilities – with an olympic sized swimming pool and tar track.
- Transport is provided for all placements, so travel expenses do not exist.

Bad things about UEA

- Constant review and refinement of the course leads to endless evaluation forms to fill in.
- Whilst most clinicians are very enthusiastic about the new curriculum, some are still determined to voice their opposition.
- Despite a small population at present, the medical school buildings can be a little crowded and groups are thrown out into obscure buildings across campus for group work.
- Car parking in the university is hard, but not impossible. Walking, cycling, and catching the bus are the best options.
- The library opening times are not great in the university, but students have 24-hour access to the hospital medical library.

Further information

The Admissions Office
School of Medicine
University of East Anglia
Norwich
Tel: 01603 591072
Fax: 01603 593752
Email: med.admiss@uea.ac.uk
Web: http://www.uea.ac.uk

Additional application information

Average A-level requirements	• AAB
Average Scottish Higher requirements	• AABB
Graduate entry requirements	• 2:1 (preferably in biological science)
Make-up of interview panel	• One academic and one clinician
Months in which interviews are held	• November–February
Proportion of overseas students	• 0%
Proportion of mature students	• No information
Proportion of graduate students	• 40%
Faculty's view of students taking a gap year	• Acceptable
Proportion of students taking intercalated degrees	• None at present
Possibility of direct entrance to clinical phase	• None
Fees for overseas students	• N/A
Fees for graduates	• £1125
Ability to transfer to other medical schools	• Owing to the unique nature of the course, it may be difficult to transfer to other schools
Assistance for elective funding	• None at present
Assistance for travel to attachments	• All transport is provided
Access and hardship funds	• Plenty of access through the main university
Weekly rent	• £45–£65, bills included for campus residences
Pint of lager	• Campus: £1.60–£1.70; city: £1.60–£2.20
Cinema	• Campus: £2.75 (or £12.50 for the year) City: £3.60–£5
Nightclub	• £2–£6

Edinburgh

Key facts	Premedical	Undergraduate
Course length	6 years	5 years
Total number of medical undergraduates	11	1280
Applicants in 2003	100	2050
Interviews given in 2003	45	
Places available in 2003	c.10	218
Places available in 2004	c.10	218
Open days 2004	mid-June	
Entrance requirements		AAAB
Mandatory subjects		Chemistry (A-level) Biology (at least AS-level)
Male:female ratio		35:65
Is an exam included in the selection process? If yes, what form does this exam take?	No	No
Qualification gained	MBChB	

Although it is one of the oldest medical schools, Edinburgh has shed the traditional preclinical/clinical course for a new integrated curriculum that started in October 1998. With a strong research tradition (reflected by 40% of students taking an intercalated BSc), Edinburgh seems to attract high academic achievers and a lot of students from England and Northern Ireland. The medical school is situated centrally, which means that you mix well with other students and feel a real part of the university and the city itself – a compact yet varied centre to escape into.

Education

The new curriculum is taught in teaching hospitals, in district general hospitals, and on attachment in GP practices. It is structured in an integrated fashion, with themes of clinical skills and communication skills running across all 5 years. Studying starts with the normal function of the body, building through to disease processes and clinical systems. Although there is some clinical involvement in the early years (particularly in general practice settings), the bulk of clinical placements are in years 3–5.

Teaching

The general trend is towards lectures and tutorials in the first couple of years, with formalised en-masse teaching being replaced by ward-based teaching later on in the course. Although there is some problem- or case-based work, most of the teaching is by formal lectures and small group sessions. These are balanced between tutorials and group work, led by facilitators, with the aim of gaining not only knowledge but also group-work skills. Anatomy is taught with prosected material and computer-assisted learning programmes.

Assessment

Exams are normally at the end of each term, count for at least 60% of the course mark, and consist of a combination of MCQ and short answer papers. In addition there is an increasing emphasis on continuous and modular assessment in the new curriculum, and students are required to build up a portfolio of essays and patient case studies, which will form the basis for part of the final assessment.

Intercalated degrees

At Edinburgh there is a well-established Honours programme and a large number of students intercalate each year. Places are dependent on a good academic performance and, whilst most students choose traditional science courses, a few places are available for subjects such as sports medicine and psychology. Each year a few students choose to study at other universities.

Special study modules and electives

Electives take place in year 5 and last for 2 months, and the faculty is very flexible about what you do and where you go – just as long as it's medically related. There are also several periods for special study modules (also called options, projects, etc) starting in small groups in years 1 and 2, and leading to an independent research project for 14 weeks in year 4. This is a great opportunity to do your own ground-breaking research in a university renowned for it!

Erasmus

There is the opportunity to study for certain intercalated BSc subjects in Leiden (Netherlands). Outside the Erasmus scheme, you are able to do your elective virtually anywhere in the world that you want, so long as the faculty approves it.

Facilities

Library There is a dedicated medical library, which is well used and is especially busy at exam times. The availability of recommended textbooks on short loan is good. It is open 9 am–10 pm

Monday to Thursday, and until 5 pm on Friday and Saturday, and 12–5 pm on Sunday afternoon. Holiday opening is until 7 pm, including during the summer break when there are still clinical students working. Most DGHs also have small libraries.

Computer facilities   There is a dedicated computer laboratory in the medical school with 100 PCs; word-processing, email, internet, and specially designed computer-assisted learning packages are available, and it is open 24 hours via a swipe card. Although it can get very busy during the day, there are more computers available in the medical library as well as the rest of the university, and many university-owned properties have computer facilities in them or on site. In the majority of hospitals outside the city there is access to the university network – however, the number of computers and the access to them varies.

Clinical skills   There are excellent clinical skills laboratories at both the main hospitals. These are very well-equipped and along with the set teaching sessions, the staff make themselves readily available to students who would like some extra coaching.

Welfare

Student support

Faculty can seem a little harsh and traditional when you first arrive. However, each student has a Director of Studies responsible for monitoring your progress and providing pastoral care, which acts as an effective safety net. Faculty tends to take a hands-off approach, which on one level gives you freedom and independence, but can leave you feeling like a small drop in a big ocean. However, if you have genuine difficulties then the faculty is extremely helpful and genuinely flexible. The faculty has good relations with the Medical Students' Council and a comprehensive *Student Handbook* is published jointly every year.

Accommodation

University accommodation in halls or flats is guaranteed in year 1. However, demand from all students for halls (which are of a good standard) is greater than the places available, and after year 1 most students get a group together and rent a flat from a private landlord or the university. Some students also choose to take out a mortgage to buy their own flats, renting rooms to other students; however, property in Edinburgh is becoming increasingly expensive. An advantage of Edinburgh is that most of the student accommodation is very central for the university and the city, and almost invariably within 15–20 minutes' walking distance. However, the cold winters do put up your heating bills.

Placements

For the first 2 years medics are a real part of the university, with the medical school being centrally placed in George Square. It is very handy for all the library facilities, computers, unions, and halls. However, now that the New Royal Infirmary is open and services are gradually being moved there, it is not yet clear how much of the medical school will remain on the university site and how much will

Location of clinical placement/name of hospital	Distance away from medical school (miles)	Difficulty getting there on public transport*	Accommodation available
New Royal Infirmary	7	+	No
Western General	5	+	No
Livingston	14	++	Yes
Dunfermline	17	++	Yes
Stirling	38	+++	Yes

*Eaoo of aoooooibility: ı, oct your alarm clock carly; ı ı, long journey; +++, car is a must

move out. It will certainly change the feel of things. In the last 3 years of the course, most time is spent in the hospitals and often away from Edinburgh, so medics can begin to lose touch with their student roots and see less of their colleagues.

In year 1 students go into general practices twice for two well-received community-based practicals. Time in year 2 is spent in local GP practices learning clinical skills. In year 3 you may have the rare clinic outside the city. In years 4 and 5 a significant amount of time is spent on blocks in peripheral hospitals up to 80 miles from Edinburgh, as well as in general practices. There are normally at least two students on the placement, and accommodation is provided free of charge. As there are fewer students you get much more involved in the team, and the teaching is generally as good as (if not better than) in central teaching hospitals. However, transport can be difficult if you don't have a car.

The two main teaching hospitals are the New Royal Infirmary and the Western General, which are both about a 25-minute bus ride away (about 80p). Both have an atmosphere of pioneering, cutting-edge medicine, and surgery. The facilities for students are adequate. There all sorts of patients to learn from and ward groups are normally small (six or seven students in year 3 – but tending to get a bit bigger – and two students per ward in years 4 and 5). If you put the effort in, you'll get a lot out of it.

Sports and social 🏆

City life

Edinburgh, the city of festivals, is a great place to spend 5 years of your life. The university is centrally placed, with the medical school at the heart of the university. Although it is the capital of Scotland, Edinburgh has more than its fair share of English and overseas residents, so there is a very cosmopolitan atmosphere. For the first 2 years you really blend into mainstream student life, but the time-consuming clinical years mean that you gradually drift away from the main student body. There is a strong community spirit within each year group, and no shortage of medic societies, sports clubs, and socialising.

Edinburgh has the advantage of being a compact and generally safe city where everything is within walking distance. It is a lively cosmopolitan capital city with a good pub and club scene, theatres, cinemas, shopping, and a lot of tourist attractions. Although it is a huge tourist trap (especially during the Military Tattoo and the International Festival and Fringe in the summer), the tourists' and students' paths don't really cross. Between the three universities there is a large student population, which is very well catered for. Edinburgh has one of the highest concentrations of pubs in a city centre, and most are licensed to 1 am (clubs open to 3 am). Green space is found at the Meadows and Holyrood Park. Both are excellent, with friendly football, rugby, hockey, American football, korfball matches, etc. Edinburgh is well connected for getting to most other parts of the UK, and the great outdoors is not too far away if you want to get away from it all for some fresh air.

University life

The Medical Students' Council, Royal Medical Society (which has rooms open 24 hours to members), and each year's final year club organise social events, talks, and balls. There is also a medics' choir and orchestra, an active Christian Medics group, and the medical school magazine *2nd Opinion*. In short, if you want it, it is probably there (and if it isn't, you can set it up)! Apart from traditional medic activities (various balls, plays, revue, academic families), most students find their own entertainment in the city itself rather than relying exclusively upon medical societies. The Union is one of the largest in the country, offers a good range of societies, and is an excellent venue. The Unions (as a group) do have lots of competition from the city itself.

Sports life

The medics' rugby team is well organised and successful, with a formidable reputation both on and off the field. A mixed hockey team and a netball team have recently been formed, and what they (sometimes) lack in skill they make up for in character. There are various year football and badminton teams. Medics tend to play a more active part in the wider university sports scene rather than just staying within the medical school. Most sports people who represent the medical school will also play for the main university and/or local clubs.

Fascinating fact: Medicine has been taught at Edinburgh since the 16th century. Two of its most famous individuals are Joseph Lister, who was the first to practise aseptic surgery, and Sir James Young Simpson, who discovered chloroform anaesthesia.

Great things about Edinburgh

- Edinburgh is a vibrant and lively university and city with excellent shopping, pubs, and clubs. The Festivals and Hogmanay are an extremely important part of the city's spirit, and the new Scottish Parliament has added to the city's cosmopolitan charms.
- BOO! Edinburgh is renowned for its ghosts and is one of the most haunted cities in the world. There are many scary and exciting tours, many of which enter into the vaults under the city!

- Edinburgh hosts a lot of innovative and world-respected research projects in clinical medicine and surgery. You will be taught by some very big names!
- You can drink in pubs and restaurants 24 hours a day if you know how (and want to).
- The medical students have a very good collective spirit, especially in the first 3 years, without being too cliquey.

Bad things about Edinburgh 👎

- Large numbers of tourists, festival luvvies, and the New Year Hogmanay invasion.
- The support network works well in a crisis, but you can feel a bit anonymous to the faculty at other times.
- Peripheral attachments in the latter years mean that the year group doesn't meet up very often.
- Without a car, travelling to peripheral hospitals can be awkward.
- It gets very cold and windy in winter.

Further information

Admissions Office
Faculty of Medicine
Medical School
Teviot Place
Edinburgh EH8 9AG
Tel: 0131 650 3187
Fax: 0131 650 6525
Email: medug@ed.ac.uk
Web: http://www.ed.ac.uk

Additional application information

Average A-level requirements	• AAAB, chemistry to A-level, plus maths, physics or biology. Biology at least to AS level. Three A-levels accepted where verified evidence student has been unable to access four subjects. Full details at www.ed.ac.uk
Average Scottish Higher requirements	• AAAAB, including chemistry, plus two out of biology, maths, and physics
Graduate entry requirements	• Minimum 2:1 (science based degree preferred). Edinburgh is happy to consider applications from graduates for the standard course
Make-up of interview panel	• Three selectors (teaching staff)
Months in which interviews are held	• December–February
Proportion of overseas students	• 7.5%
Proportion of mature students	• 5%
Proportion of graduate students	• 10%
Faculty's view of students taking a gap year	• Entirely happy if put to educational use
Proportion of students taking intercalated degrees	• 40%
Possibility of direct entrance to clinical phase	• Yes
Fees for overseas students	• £10 000 pa (preclinical) £19 000 pa (clinical)
Fees for graduates	• See Chapter 6
Ability to transfer to other medical schools	• Unusual, however special circumstances will be considered by the faculty
Assistance for elective funding	• Funding and advice are available through various organisations such as the Royal Medical Society
Assistance for travel to attachments	• Free buses run between city hospitals. No other assistance from medical school
Access and hardship funds	• Available. Enquire through tutor system
Weekly rent	• £45–£80. Depends how up-market your flat is
Pint of lager	• £1.50–£3.00. Depends whether you just want a pint or want to be seen! Plenty of pubs
Cinema	• £3.50–£5.50
Nightclub	• £0–£8. Huge variety. Every taste catered for

Glasgow

Key facts	Undergraduate
Course length	5 years
Total number of medical undergraduates	c 1200
Applicants in 2003	1321
Interviews given in 2003	850
Places available in 2003	241
Places available in 2004	241
Open days 2004	8 September
Entrance requirements	AAB
Mandatory subjects	Chemistry (and biology if Highers)
Male:female ratio	36:64
Is an exam included in the selection process? If yes, what form does this exam take?	No
Qualification gained	MBChB

Glasgow medical school has its historical origins in the 17th century and is a well-renowned centre for teaching and research excellence, particularly for cardiovascular disease and cancer. It is currently housed in the newly opened Wolfson Medical School Building situated on the main university campus. As with nearly all medical curricula in the UK, Glasgow has undergone some changes to fulfil the GMC requirements and expectations of tomorrow's doctor.

Education

The new problem-based learning course is now in its 8th year and has achieved a fine balance between teaching vocational and scientific aspects and equipping the modern student with the skills they need to embark upon the ever-changing world of a career in medicine.

Teaching

The mainstay of the course is problem-based learning (PBL) sessions. These involve groups of 10 students, guided by a facilitator, tackling two medical scenarios each week. There are also some supporting laboratory (fixed resource sessions) and lectures (plenaries). A week of lectures at the beginning of the both years 2 and 3 have now also been introduced to give students a better scientific grounding before they embark on their PBL sessions.

The traditional preclinical/clinical divide has been eroded to some extent – patient contact and practical skills are now taught from week 1. However, the bulk of hospital-based teaching still takes place in years 4 and 5.

Assessment

Continuous assessment in the form of essays takes place in every 5-week block in years 1 and 2. Two formal written exams on all aspects of the work covered are taken at the end of year 1, along with an additional exam testing a student's ability to work through a problem. This is known as the medical independent learning exam (MILE) in which a scenario is handed out with a set of pertinent questions, which a student has 24 hours to work through. From year 2 onwards objective structured clinical exams (OSCE) form part of the assessment process.

Years 4 and 5 are treated as a continuum consisting of 10 x 5-week blocks: three in medicine and surgery and one in General Practice, Child Health, Obstetrics and Gynaecology, and Psychiatry. Although there are no exams until the end of year 5, the student's allocated block supervisor must assess as to whether he/she has passed the block; if not, it will need to be repeated.

Intercalated degrees

There are both 1- and 2-year intercalated degree options: 1-year courses are available in clinical or science subjects and lead to a BSc MedSci (Hons); the 2-year BSc (Hons) option is available only in science subjects. The intercalated degree courses are undertaken between years 3 and 4.

Special study modules and electives

Special study modules cover a wide range of subjects and constitute about 20% of the overall course time. There is one 5-week block in second year, and two in each year thereafter. Students choose from a list of options and may propose their own from year 3 onwards. Almost any topic can be studied, including non-medical subjects such as French or philosophy, and SSMs can be taken abroad in years 3, 4, and 5. There are two 4-week electives during the summers of the years 3 and 4, which can also be spent abroad. In some circumstances, an SSM can be amalgamated with an elective to provide a greater depth of study in a topic of interest.

Erasmus

There is currently no ERASMUS programme at Glasgow. However, the many opportunities to travel abroad for SSMs and electives, make Glasgow one of the best universities in which to study if overseas opportunities are a priority.

Facilities

Library   The main university library, with an excellent range of reference books and journals, is open until 11 pm on weekdays and during the day at weekends. The new medical school building includes a purpose-built "study landscape" well equipped with books and journals. Additional study facilities are available on campus (24 hours in Unions) and in all hospitals, some of which are open 24 hours. The new building also has three floors of extensive library and computing facilities along with smaller seminar rooms, which can be booked for group study.

Computers   There is good central provision of computers in the main university library, with over 300 PCs available. The medical school study landscape provides over 100 flat-screen multimedia PCs that allow students to access a range of electronic learning facilities. Facilities are increasing and improving all the time, with about 20 PCs available for students in each of the main teaching hospitals, and peripheral hospitals gradually being linked to the campus network.

Clinical skills   Students are taught clinical skills from year 1, including first aid and basic/advanced resuscitation. The new medical school building includes a fully equipped ward and side rooms containing audiovisual facilities to enable students to study their own performance in a simulated clinical environment before being confronted with a real hospital situation. Other new facilities include a cardiology patient simulator (known as Harvey), which can mimic symptoms of up to 26 cardiac diseases.

Welfare

Student support

Glasgow is renowned for its friendly and relaxed atmosphere, and the medical school is no exception. Each student is allocated an Adviser of Studies to offer advice and support, and most tutors are very approachable. The Medico-Chirurgical (the medics' own society) operates a "Mums and Dads" scheme for freshers with second-years acting as parents to guide the new first-year intake! Glasgow has the usual university counselling and welfare services including a telephone nightline open from 7 pm to 7 am every night, operated by the Students' Representative Council.

Accommodation

Glasgow has a large number of local students, but it tries to guarantee accommodation to first-year students moving to the city, and 35% of hall places are reserved for returning students. The vast majority of these places are in catered halls of residence. The university has little control over private sector flats but there is an accommodation office to help you. Average rents are £65 per week for full board in halls, £40 (plus bills) per week for a 52-week lease on a university flat, and £45–£65 (plus bills) per week for private flats.

Placements

Glasgow has a large, attractive campus in the west end of the city, 2 miles from the centre. Six large teaching hospitals within the Glasgow area and 13 district general hospitals (DGHs) provide the mainstay of the teaching. The teaching hospitals used include the Glasgow Royal Infirmary, the Western Infirmary, Gartnavel, and Stobhill Hospitals. Some of the DGHs used are some distance away, but free accommodation is provided and the facilities (although not quite the London Hilton) are clean and warm. Groups of students number between five and eight. This drops to two per ward by the final year.

For placements outside the university, peripheral attachments can take you to Paisley (8 miles) or as far as Dumfries (80 miles). However, there are many hospitals and general practices in the Greater Glasgow area and GP practices are likely to be local.

Location of clinical placement/name of hospital	Distance away from medical school (miles)	Difficulty getting there on public transport*	Accommodation available
Royal Alexandra (Paisley)	8	+	No
Hairmyres	13	++	No
Monklands	20	++	Yes
Wishaw	20	++	No
Crosshouse	30	+++	Yes
Ayr	40	++	Yes
Inverclyde	30	+++	Yes
Dumfries	80	+++	Yes
Stirling	30	++	Yes
Falkirk	35	+++	Yes
Vale of Leven	30	+++	No
Ravenscraig	30	+++	No

*Ease of accessibility: +, set your alarm clock early; ++, long journey; +++, car is a must

Sports and social 🏆

City life

Glasgow is Scotland's biggest city and is truly international, with a large city centre containing all that you would expect to find. The main university buildings are among Glasgow's landmarks, with beautiful architecture and real atmosphere. The Gilbert Scott tower, the main university spire, is one of the highest points in the city. There is lots of student accommodation in flats in the west end close to the university, and near to great pubs, shops, and a lively club scene.

Glasgow was the 1999 City of Art and Design and 1990 European City of Culture, which reflects its interesting architecture and design history, and cultural past and present. You are never short of something to do or see in Glasgow, from the well-established Kelvingrove Gallery (currently undergoing refurbishment due to open in 2006), which houses one of the best art collections in the UK, to the new Museum of Modern Art. Glasgow also boasts some of the best shopping in Scotland (including over 40 shops in the new city centre Buchanan Galleries) and a leading club/pub scene. Not for you? How about an Old Firm game: Glasgow has the two largest Scottish football teams and many first-division rugby sides. The city also hosts many international athletic events. If you want a change of scene, getting out of Glasgow is easy enough, with access to some of the best hill walking, climbing, and skiing in the UK, a mere 1–2 hours away. Other Scottish cities are also close at hand, with Edinburgh and the new Parliament only 45 minutes away. Buses and trains leave every 15 minutes.

University life

The Medico-Chirurgical Society (Med-Chir) is an educational and social society set up and run by medical students. It meets every Thursday, with free beer and talks from a range of speakers on a variety of entertaining topics. It also arranges events, including trips abroad, the annual ball, the annual revue, and a musical culture night. Each year has its own year club to organise club nights, ceilidhs, and balls, and to raise money for a massive graduation ball. Our medical students' magazine *Surgo* will also keep you updated on all the activities and gossip within the faculty. Unusually, Glasgow has two Unions: Glasgow University Union (GUU) and Queen Margaret Union (QMU), both with bars, clubs, catering facilities, and a regular programme of bands, balls, and special events. The GUU has a Debating Chamber and Glasgow University has won the World Debating Championships more times than any other university. All the usual (and some unusual) clubs and societies are available for students to join.

Sports life

The sports centre at the heart of the campus has recently undergone a massive refurbishment programme. The facilities include a 25-m pool, sauna, weights room, squash courts, and sports hall. For only £20 per year you can have unlimited access to the sports facilities, as well as a wide range of daily classes in aerobics, muscle conditioning, and circuits. There is also a large off-campus sports facility housing tennis courts, floodlit hockey and football pitches, and another new gym. There are a variety of sports clubs on offer, from football and rugby through to swimming, squash, canoeing, and horse riding. Med-Chir also has medics' football and rugby teams.

Fascinating fact: Dr Ian McDonald – pioneer of the ultrasound – and the neurosurgeon Professor Graham Teasdale, who is responsible for the Glasgow Coma Scale (used worldwide), are both famous medics linked to Glasgow.

Great things about Glasgow 👍

- Prime west end location; lots of shops, cafés, and restaurants.
- Great facilities: two great Unions, sports complex, main library, and a well-equipped new medical school building.
- Large number of teaching hospitals.
- Teaching by internationally acclaimed experts.
- Chance to mix with students from all corners of the world.

Bad things about Glasgow 👎

- The weather: bring a brolley!
- Some of the district hospitals are far away.
- Little contact with students from other courses.
- Lack of free parking in and around the university and central hospitals.
- Vehicle congestion especially in city centre and west end.

Further information

Admissions Enquiries
Wolfson Medical School
University of Glasgow
University Avenue
Glasgow G12 8QQ
Tel: 0141 330 6216
Fax: 0141 330 2776
Email: admissions@clinmed.gla.ac.uk
Web: www.medicine.gla.ac.uk

Additional application information

Average A-level requirements	• AAB (at first attempt) in chemistry and at least one from biology, maths or physics
Average Scottish Higher requirements	• AAAAB in year 5. Chemistry and biology plus one of maths and physics
Graduate entry requirements	• 2:1 in any discipline. If the degree is non-science, science based A-levels or Highers are required, completed within the last 5 years
Make-up of interview panel	• Two doctors
Months in which interviews are held	• November–March
Proportion of overseas students	• 7.5%
Proportion of mature students	• Various by year – no quota
Proportion of graduate students	• 15%
Faculty's view of students taking a gap year	• Acceptable if used constructively
Proportion of students taking intercalated degrees	• 30%
Possibility of direct entrance to clinical phase	• No
Fees for overseas students	• £16 500 pa
Fees for graduates	• See Chapter 6
Ability to transfer to other medical schools	• The Faculty is usually keen to avoid this, unless it is in the format of an intercalated degree, which is not offered in Glasgow
Assistance for elective funding	• The faculty invites students to apply for help with costs they might incur during their elective. However, only one application for funding a junior or senior elective is considered from each student
Assistance for travel to attachments	• Available to some students through LEA/ELB/SAAS
Access and hardship funds	• Some money available from the faculty for postgraduate students. There are also university wide hardship funds, which all students can access if they are in need
Weekly rent	• £55
Pint of lager	• £1.60
Cinema	• £3.50
Nightclub	• Usually free entry but some may charge up to £3

Glasgow

Guy's, King's, and St Thomas'

Key facts	Premedical	Undergraduate	Graduate
Course length	6 years	5 years	4 years
Total number of medical undergraduates	40	1800	40
Applicants in 2003	365	3300	N/A
Interviews given in 2003	115	1200	N/A
Places available in 2003	40	360	N/A
Places available in 2004	40	320	40
Open days 2004	July	July	TBA
Entrance requirements		ABB/C	2:1 any discipline
Mandatory subjects	None	Chemistry + biology	None
Male:female ratio	32:67	35:64	–
Is an exam included in the selection process? If yes, what form does this exam take?	No	No	Yes, MSAT
Qualification gained	MBBS		

Guy's, King's, and St Thomas' School of Medicine, popularly known as GKT, was formed in August 1998 by the merger of the United Medical and Dental School (UMDS) of Guy's and St Thomas' Hospitals and King's College School of Medicine and Dentistry (KCSMD). It is part of King's College London.

The school combines two established medical schools, both with long histories, including older mergers: King's College is a multidisciplinary institution, part of the University of London, and had its own medical school at King's College Hospital in south London. Guy's and St Thomas' Hospitals had their own medical schools prior to the merger to form the United Medical and Dental Schools.

An intake of nearly 400 students makes the new school one of the biggest medical schools in the UK, and King's College as a whole the largest centre for healthcare teaching in Europe. Both King's and GKT emphasise personal academic development (for example, a strongly supported intercalated BSc programme) and encourage students to participate fully in extracurricular activities.

Education

The course is split into two main sections of which the first 2 years place an emphasis on the basic medical sciences. There is early clinical contact, with communication teaching taking place in a GP setting from year 1. The course is organised into systems, for example cardiovascular or musculoskeletal. All the core basic science teaching takes place at the Guy's Hospital campus.

Clinical disciplines are taught in the latter 3 years on the wards of St Thomas' Hospital, King's College Hospital, Guy's Hospital, University Hospital Lewisham, and also in the community. The long-established systems-based clinical course has been designed to complement the course structure from the earlier years. The core clinical subjects are delivered and examined during years 3 and 4. The final year consists of an 8-week elective, followed by attachments in the community and attachments shadowing medical and surgical house officers in district general hospitals.

Teaching

Teaching is conducted via a mixture of lectures, tutorials, and practicals, mixed in with computer-assisted learning. Dissection is still a valued part of preclinical teaching.

Assessment

Essay and short-answer questions are now rare during years 3–5. Written examinations during the clinical years are mostly computer marked, and offer some element of choice in the answer. OSCEs (objective structured clinical exams) are the main practical examinations during the clinical years, starting with a short communication skills OSCE in year 2.

Intercalated degrees

There are well-supported intercalated degree programmes at the college. These include a wide range of subjects, including some outside medicine. Students can also choose to study for their intercalated degree at alternative London colleges or other UK universities.

Special study modules and electives

About 20% of each year is devoted to SSMs. There is a considerable range of subjects available and the number is increasing every year. As the school is part of a multifaculty institution there are also many non-medical SSMs available, such as a choice of modern languages and the popular history of medicine. In addition, students are free to design their own SSM if the subject they wish to study is not on offer.

The 8-week elective period is an opportunity to travel to far-flung destinations (or just down the road) to study in fields of medicine of your choosing. There is some assessment of how time is spent on the elective (to discourage the temptation to just lie on a beach for 12 weeks), in the form of a poster presentation. Various awards and sponsorships are available to help students fund their electives.

Erasmus

Despite the end of GKT participation in ERASMUS schemes, the school has special links with numerous medical schools around the world, including the Johns Hopkins University in the USA, the University of Hong Kong, the University of West Indies, and Moscow Medical Academy. As GKT is twinned with these institutions, there are special allocations for GKT students who want to do their electives there. Accommodation will also usually be arranged and extra bursaries may be available to help with travel costs to these colleges.

Added opportunities

Access to Medicine is a major initiative to widen access to medical degree courses. The programme is specifically designed to help bright and talented young people from backgrounds associated with low aspirations to become doctors. The programme will eventually allow for up to 50 extra undergraduate places in medicine and will be for talented school pupils from south London who would not normally achieve the necessary grades to train as doctors. The course is based on a standard MBBS course but will take 6 years rather than 5, because of the addition of special modules in the first 3 years.

Facilities

Library   Libraries at Guy's are open between 9 am and 9 pm on weekdays, 9 am and 5 pm on Saturday, and 1 pm and 5 pm on Sunday; there is also a large 24-hour study room. At King's College Hospital the library is open until 9 pm on weekdays and 1 pm on Saturday. Students also have access to the King's College London library at the old Public Records Office in Chancery Lane, which is open until 9 pm from Monday to Thursday, 6 pm on Friday, and 5.30 pm on Saturday and Sunday. All libraries have a good range of books and journals.

Computers   All campuses have a large number of computer stations with access to email, the internet, and computer-assisted learning programs designed in-house. There are 24-hour computing facilities at Guy's, and late/weekend opening at the St Thomas' campus. The "virtual campus" is a specialised area of the King's College London website for the GKT Schools of Medicine, Dentistry, and Biomedical Sciences and enables students to do things like download lecture notes, register for course components, or obtain details (but not the answers) about their exams.

Clinical skills   A new clinical skills centre opened at Guy's in 1999. It is the largest of its kind in Europe, and is available every weekday from 9 am to 5 pm. Students can book individual rooms in small groups or with their tutor. There are also various laboratories at the three main hospitals. These are great places, with latex models of every imaginable part of the human anatomy on which students can practise their clinical skills, such as taking blood pressure or suturing – in the past, King's students on A&E attachments practised suturing pigs' trotters before being let loose on the population of south London!

Welfare

Student support

Students are assigned to a personal tutor to support them throughout the course. Welfare and counselling services are available on the Guy's campus, where there is a welfare officer available every day. All sites are friendly environments with lots of support from the faculty and staff, as well as the Student Union who provide student representation over a wide range of matters. The Student Medical Education Committee (SMEC) is a unique student committee that is actively involved in course development and provides feedback to course organisers on how things are going. It acts as a dedicated link between the medical school and the student body. There are six elected representatives in each year, and they will help students to deal with any problems that arise with the course, and address any associated welfare concerns.

Accommodation

College accommodation is available in many different parts of London. Some residences may be on or near the campuses themselves (on-site accommodation is available on the Guy's campus), whereas others may be much further away. The quality and cost of private accommodation can vary a lot in the central Guy's/St Thomas' area, but cheaper, good-quality accommodation is more readily available in the Denmark Hill area. Students can opt for Intercollegiate University of London accommodation, although these tend to be some distance from any of the campuses.

Placements

Students in years 1 and 2 are taught at the Guy's Hospital campus at London Bridge. The campus is shared with other departments in biomedical sciences and dentistry. A large new building houses most of the above disciplines, with state-of-the-art library and computing facilities. Most of the clinical teaching takes place at St Thomas' Hospital, King's College Hospital, Guy's Hospital, and University Hospital Lewisham. Students can also access King's College's other campuses, including the Strand campus and Waterloo campus. Guy's, St Thomas', and the Strand campuses are all situated within a square mile on both sides of the Thames in central London. Psychiatry teaching takes place at the Maudsley Hospital and the Institute of Psychiatry, which has been awarded the status of 5-star top research institute in the UK.

As well as the central teaching hospitals in years 4 and 5, there are placements in district general hospitals in southeast England. This relieves some of the pressures at the central London teaching hospitals and provides access to high-quality teaching; clinical workloads tend to be lower, and consultants are able to devote more time to students.

Location of clinical placement/name of hospital	Distance away from medical school (miles)	Difficulty getting there on public transport*	Accommodation available
Woolwich	5	+	No
Bromley	8	+	No
Canterbury	30	++	Yes
Brighton	50	+++	Yes
Salisbury	90	+++	Yes

*Ease of accessibility: +, set your alarm clock early; ++, long journey; +++, car is a must

Sports and social 🏆

City life

Most of the campuses are close to the centre of London, with all of London's attractions within easy reach by public transport.

University life

The old colleges always had thriving social scenes, with numerous balls, weekly events, the annual revues, and arguably the best university Divali Show and Rag week. There is a vast selection of clubs and societies to join, including orchestras, bands, singing, dancing, drama and musical theatre groups; everyone can usually find something that interests them, or comrades with which to start up a new society. The Students' Union run our very own bars, shops, cafés, nightclubs, and gym. Student bars are present on all campuses, and there is the main college nightclub at the Strand campus. If all that's not enough, all students have access to the University of London Union (ULU) with its own range of facilities.

GKT gives students access to a large multidisciplinary institution while retaining the friendliness of a medical school. With its almost enclosed courtyard, promenade, and grass park at London Bridge, the Guy's campus is regarded as the closest thing to a campus university in central London. Multifaith pastoral care is provided on all campuses, and there are many student-run religious groups covering the main religious faiths. The mix of students on a day-to-day basis may not be diverse, but as students use King's College and University of London Union facilities there will be plenty of opportunity for integration. Students are also encouraged to get involved in Community Action volunteering programmes, working with homeless and disadvantaged people within the local area.

Sports life

Particularly strong sports include rugby, football, hockey, netball, tennis, badminton, rowing, and squash, alongside the oldest rugby team in the world at Guy's. There is also a strong tradition of karate. GKT has sports grounds at Honor Oak Park in south London, Dulwich, and Cobham in Surrey, giving facilities for rugby, football, and hockey. King's College also has sports grounds in Surbiton. There are gyms at the Guy's and St Thomas' campuses, and also at the Stamford Street halls of residence. For swimmers, there is a pool at Guy's.

Fascinating fact: Guy's Hospital, with its 30-storey "tower" boasting spectacular views over London, holds the record of being the tallest hospital in the world.

Great things about GKT

- GKT hospitals are all world renowned.
- Excellent range of learning and social facilities at the medical school campuses.
- The school is part of a multifaculty institution. Students have the opportunity to mix with a variety of students from other courses, and have access to a wide range of facilities.
- Good sports clubs.
- Welfare and student support mechanisms are well established and are effective.

Bad things about GKT

- Cost of living in London.
- Student accommodation can be a long way from your campus.
- Large number of medics in each year group can lead to it being a bit impersonal.
- Clinical placements can be quite far away and expensive to travel to.
- The medical school can be a bit bureaucratic.

Further information

Student Admissions Officer
The Hodgkin Building
Guy's Hospital Campus
King's College London
St Thomas' Street
London Bridge
London SE1 9RT
Tel: 020 7848 6501/6502
Fax: 020 7848 6510
Email: gktadmissions@kcl.ac.uk
Web: http://www.kcl.ac.uk

Additional application information

Average A-level requirements	• ABB/C, including chemistry and biology (at least one to A-level and one to AS-level) at first attempt
Average Scottish Higher requirements	• Only accept Highers for 6-year programme AAABB in any five subjects. Advanced Highers accepted for 5-year programme. Contact admissions for exact requirements
Graduate entry requirements	• 2:1 in any discipline
Make-up of interview panel	• Two, comprising academics, clinicians
Months in which interviews are held	• November–April (March for graduate course)
Proportion of overseas students	• 7.5%
Proportion of mature students	• 16%
Proportion of graduate students	• 16%
Faculty's view of students taking a gap year	• Encouraged
Proportion of students taking intercalated degrees	• 50%
Possibility of direct entrance to clinical phase	• Yes
Fees for overseas students	• c £13 000 (preclinical) c £23 000 (clinical)
Fees for graduates	• See Chapter 6
Ability to transfer to other medical schools	• Yes, for Intercalated BSc or for clinical years
Assistance for elective funding	• Good – both college awards and advice for external sources
Assistance for travel to attachments	• No – and some attachments are far away
Access and hardship funds	• Excellent student support and hardship facilities
Weekly rent	• £80 (London prices!)
Pint of lager	• £2.00 upward
Cinema	• £5 upward
Nightclub	• Free–£15

Hull and York

Key facts	Undergraduate
Course length	5 years
Total number of medical undergraduates	130
Applicants in 2003	1100 (2003 entry) 1650 (2004 entry)
Interviews given in 2003	700
Places available in 2003	130
Places available in 2004	130
Open days 2004	York: 5 July and 7 October Hull: 3 July and 25 September
Entrance requirements	AAB (excluding general studies)
Mandatory subjects	Chemistry and biology (one to A-level one to AS-level)
Male:female ratio	3.5:6.5
Is an exam included in the selection process? If yes, what form does this exam take?	No
Qualification gained	MBBS

September 2003 saw the long awaited opening of the Hull York Medical School (HYMS) and its first 136 students take up their places on a new and hugely exciting programme of medical education. HYMS is a collaboration between the long established and well-respected universities of Hull and York. Both universities have a wealth of experience in health and bioscience education and the medical school is very much a natural progression in their development.

HYMS is forward looking. Its aim is not only to accommodate the growing need for doctors in the UK but also to set the pace in delivering a curriculum and education that will equip them for the realities of 21st-century practice and ensure that they truly are "Tomorrow's Doctors".

Education

Students are divided equally between two campuses at Hull and York universities. Despite the physical separation for years 1 and 2, staff and students work hard to ensure complete continuity in teaching, resources, timetables, and, indeed, social activities at the respective locations. Both locations have new custom-built facilities and the constant movement of faculty between the two locations guarantees that students have good access to all members. The running of parallel timetables and employment of moderators assures HYMS students receive the same education and opportunities regardless of where they are placed. It is desirable that the students feel integrated as, in years 3, 4, and 5, Hull and York groups combine and together follow a programme of community and hospital-based study in centres throughout east and north Yorkshire and northern Lincolnshire.

The course content is organised around the study of body systems like the reproductive, cardiovascular, and musculoskeletal systems. The 5-year course is divided into three phases. In phase I (years 1 and 2), basic sciences are studied in the context of clinical medicine. In phase II (years 3 and 4) the course becomes multicentred with teaching in hospitals, general practices, and community placements across north and east Yorkshire and northern Lincolnshire. Clinical teachers here deliver the programme and students will benefit from low student–teacher ratios and plenty of opportunity for hands-on learning in hospital and primary care settings.

Phase III, year 5 and the preregistration year, gives students extensive clinical experience in medicine, surgery, and general practice. After graduation, in the "preregistration year", close supervision and educational support continues.

Teaching

The curriculum at HYMS is designed to make education interesting and exciting. In the first 2 years, basic sciences are studied. Weekly patient case studies are used as a framework in which to conceptualise and explore the science. Clinical placements at the end of each week provide opportunity to transpose the theory into medical realities.

A broad range of learning methods are used at HYMS to meet the variety of learning objectives set by the curriculum. The focus is on flexibility and the availability of resources is as important as timetabled sessions with them. Methods include problem-based (PBL) and self-directed learning, lectures, and a staff supported resource laboratory, which contains visual aids such as anatomical models, x rays, and computer packages. Clinically orientated PBL facilitators and speakers alleviate the limitations of medical textbooks in gaining a real view of medical problems and their treatments. A new anatomy museum provides use of prosections. Typically, a lecture is delivered by a speaker at either Hull or York and beamed into the other end by an impressive video conferencing link. Technological teething problems have now all but subsided and likewise, stage fright, as students across campuses regularly engage in discussion via the video system.

At HYMS, patient contact is made from day one. Clinical placements start from the beginning of year 1 with weekly half-day attachments within a small group. In year 2, a full day per week is spent with patients, and in the second and third phases clinical experience becomes much more intense with the majority of the final year spent on placements. The early placements are arranged not only to make the science and transition to the role of doctor easier, but also to supplement several of the curriculum themes in highlighting the responsibilities and duties that come with such a position. The importance of engaging with your patient and considering the psychological and social effects of their illnesses is given strong emphasis at HYMS and reflected in the fully integrated course where complementary disciplines are learned together.

Assessment

Assessment addresses the "learning outcomes" of each stage of the course using a combination of factual tests; multiple choice questions (MCQs), modified essay and short answer, and practical patient-based assessments. Exams are conducted at the end of the summer term. Students also keep a computer-held portfolio of learning and reflective writing as a record of progress. Formative assessments – self test papers and examinations to assist learning but not included in the final degree – take place at the beginning of the summer and spring terms. These help students to recognise their strengths and weaknesses and to guide their work objectives accordingly.

Intercalated degrees

Selected students may devote an optional year, usually between phases I and II to study for an honours degree in the biomedical or health sciences or another appropriate scientific subject of their choice.

Special study Modules and electives

Special study modules provide an exciting opportunity to pursue new interests or develop existing ones. Comprising about a third of the course, they are highly valued by HYMS students and can cover a broad range of disciplines. These could be basic or social sciences, medical specialities or non-medical subjects such as languages or the arts.

The elective is an opportunity to see any medical speciality in any part of the world and takes place during phase III.

Erasmus

There is no opportunity to participate in an Erasmus programme, although students can travel abroad for their elective.

Facilities

Both Hull and York have custom-built or modified buildings and bear testimony to a substantial budget well spent. Within the buildings are the PBL rooms, which constitute the students' favourite resource. All who see them agrees: we are spoilt. Students are divided into groups of eight for problem-based learning sessions and allocated a PBL room which contains a high-tech, networked computer for each group member, a large and incredibly useful array of interactive learning packages, wall-to-wall white boards, and, most importantly, the learning support of peers in your group. Friendships and learning relationships develop quickly and strongly within these groups. PBL members have access to their own room from 6 am to 11 pm. This is where the students do the majority of their study, securing its place as a respected learning environment, a source of note-sharing, and, rumour has it, a frequent place for pizza delivery for those working late into the night.

Library The library resources are abundant and joint access to both the Hull and York libraries, regardless of your campus placement, translates to access to over 2 million books. This is before the surrounding hospital and local affiliated libraries are considered! There is a substantial collection of medical and health-related books, papers, and periodicals at both universities. Students also have access to a large number of electronic journals, multimedia CDs, videos, and the Cochrane database. At York, the medical library is part of the university's JB Morrell library. Term time opening hours are from 9 am to 10 pm and weekends from 11 am to 6 pm. Hull's Brymore Jones library opens for over 80 hours a week with excellent weekend and late night access.

Computers The medical students have in addition to the HYMS buildings, full use and 24-hour access to other computing resources across both Hull and York campuses. University and HYMS email accounts are provided. IT training and language courses are open to students at both campuses.

York runs an excellent information literacy course, ILIAD, the Languages for All Programme, enabling students to learn a foreign language whilst studying for their degree; two vocational skills-based programmes, and the York award. The latter comprises a range of courses designed to improve students' employability of which the ILIAD and Languages for All can be a component.

Hull gives all students the opportunity to develop or gain language skills and hosts the Language Institute; one of the largest and best equipped learning centres in Britain.

Clinical skills A clinical skills laboratory designed to mimic a real hospital ward provides the equipment and simulated environment in which to practice clinical techniques.

Welfare

Student support

Student welfare and a caring supportive environment are at the heart of HYMS's ethos. We are acutely aware that the most valuable commodity we have is each other, and a formidable support network comes from fellow students and the academic support gained by close contact with staff.

In addition to departmental and academic support, both Hull and York offer a range of specialist services. At the beginning of term you are introduced to the support facilities rather than having to seek them out when you need them most. These include chaplains, counselling staff, health professionals, and disability services. York has the added bonus of strong support via the College network and all HYMS welfare services are supplemented by the welfare work of the student's union.

Accommodation

Accommodation is guaranteed for all medical students at both campuses. Most students are offered rooms in halls of residence on campus; however, there are a small number of off-campus places within easy reach of the medical school. Students are able to indicate which hall they would prefer

Location of clinical placement/name of hospital	Distance away from medical school (miles)	Difficulty getting there on public transport*	Accommodation available
York NHS Services Trust	York students 2.4	+	No
Hull Royal Infirmary	Hull students 3.9	+	No
Castle Hill Hospital Hull	Hull students 9.4	++	No
Primary and secondary care placements near three partner hospitals	Near to medical schools	Various	No

*Ease of accessibility: +, set your alarm clock early; ++, long journey; +++, car is a must

to be in on their application form. Accommodation ranges from £47 to £80 per week depending on which hall you are in.

Placements

Clinical placements start from the beginning of year 1 with weekly half-day attachments within a small group. These attachments increase in frequency and duration throughout the course. In years 3, 4, and 5, Hull and York groups combine, and together follow a programme of community and hospital-based study in centres throughout east and north Yorkshire and northern Lincolnshire as part of the regional placement programme. Accommodation is provided during regional placements by the Trust where your home base is. Accommodation is not provided for students during years 1 and 2 as the partner hospitals are all in close proximity to the medical school. Students are placed at sites near their campus in years 1 and 2.

Sports and social

City life

Hull, once a hideout for beatniks and intellectuals, is now a living catwalk for the super cool and the terminally trendy. Indeed, Hull is now the focus of a recent multimillion urban regeneration project. Unfortunately, Hull suffers from preconceptions, which are far wide of the mark. Students love to live and study here. Graduates gush with praise and fondness, and the new HYMS intake are already displaying ferocious loyalty and affection for the place. The nightlife at Hull is nothing short of legendary, with numerous venues in the city centre and its very own on-campus nightclub recently voted the best university venue in the UK. Hull is unbelievable value for money. Lower accommodation costs will be difficult to come by at another university and, if you are coming from London, expect another three pints for your fiver!

Hull University holds a global reputation not only for academia, but also its friendliness. Its graduates are consistently among the top 10 UK universities for graduate employment and it places strong emphasis on students excelling both in and out of the classroom.

York is a beautiful city. Steeped in history and encircled by ancient walls, York boasts some remarkable architecture including its landmark Minster, the largest Gothic cathedral in Northern Europe, and winding medieval streets. A strong tourist industry ensures it bustles with life throughout the year and hosts a remarkable array of shops, restaurants, pubs, bistros, and sights. York has a distinctly cosmopolitan feel, catering for every interest. The Theatre Royal, Grand Opera House, and a wide variety of live music venues enrich the staple student regimen of clubs and kebabs. The university has a collegiate system; ensuring friendships can run far beyond the medical school. Socialising tends to take place in the college bars or the city centre, but York's proximity to Leeds and Manchester ensures that there are bigger nights out not too far away.

Hull and York are both couched in some of the most spectacular countryside in England. Surrounded by the Pennines, Dales, North Yorkshire Moors, and the seaside towns of Whitby, Robin Hood's Bay, and Scarborough, the area offers many opportunities for exploration. York also has the advantage of being placed half-way between Edinburgh and London, which are less than 2 hours away by train. The regular and cheap ferries running from Hull to Amsterdam require little promotion.

University life

With the array of extra curricular opportunities existing between Hull and York and HYMS, our social calendars require some organising. The enthusiastic "Medsoc", a body of eight students from both campuses who arrange events ranging from visiting speakers to charity pub-crawls, organises this. Enthusiasm and talent is not in short supply and all students are working hard to bring to life plans for unisex sports teams, a medics band, a Christmas review, and a HYMS newspaper. As a new school, clubs and projects are evolving to reflect students' interests and talents, and we eagerly await the new intake to supplement and enrich the current stream of activity.

Links with the BMA and other medical schools are growing, and HYMS is eager to establish itself in the wider community of medical students and health professionals. HYMS has been shown a warm welcome by York Medical Society and the local trust. Outside lectures, close contact is maintained between both students and staff by the web-based discussion boards and regular social activities.

Common rooms provide a place for a coffee, chat, or break, and are great for socialising.

Sports life

The sporting facilities at Hull are excellent with gyms, jacuzzis, an astroturf and squash courts. The Athletic Union currently has around 50 different sporting clubs. A magnificent new sports stadium and "The Deep", an innovative ocean discovery centre, are just two of the exciting new developments marking out the future face of the city. At York, there is an abundance of facilities, accommodating the golfer, cyclist, swimmer, climber, gym fanatic, and hardened gambler – we do have one of the finest racecourses in the country!

Fascinating fact: Dr Menos Lagopoulos and Professor Paul O'Higgins, both eminent tutors in anatomy, work at HYMS.

Great things about Hull and York

- You are spoilt with the huge amount of resources available to students.
- Clinical placements from the very beginning of the course are invaluable.
- Hull's Asylum nightclub was voted the best student union venue in the UK.
- Dr Menos Lagopoulos and Professor Paul O'Higgins our eminent tutors in anatomy. They are an unmissable double act.
- The students – HYMS is a close community where a culture of cooperation not competition reigns

Bad things about Hull and York

- With free taxis and buses put on for access to our clinical placements, will we ever adapt to public transport again?
- Self-directed and problem-based learning requires adaptation from A-level style syllabus and teaching.
- Although students get to state a preference for the campus they would like to be placed at, allocation is largely by ballot. Only exceptionally are individual personal circumstances taken into account.
- Student and staff refusal to accept that the video link is not TV and, no, your mum cannot see you wave. Will the novelty ever wear off?
- The consequences of freshers' week, or to be more specific, three freshers' weeks, are far reaching. Hull starts term a little earlier than York does and HYMS fits into the former's timetable. What this translates to is a freshers' week at HYMS, one at Hull University, and a later one at York University.

Further information

Admissions and Schools Liaison
University of York
Heslington
York YO10 5DD
Tel: 01904 321 690
Fax: 01904 321 696
Email: admissions@york.ac.uk
Web: http://www.hyms.ac.uk

Student Recruitment and Admissions Service
University of Hull
Kingston upon Hull
Hull HU6 7RX
Tel: 01482 466 497
Email: admissions@hull.ac.uk
Web: http://www.hyms.ac.uk

Additional application information

Average A-level requirements	• ABB, including chemistry or biology (minimum one at A-level grade A, one at AS-level grade B). General studies not accepted
Average Scottish Higher requirements	• AAAAB including biology and chemistry, one of which at Advanced Higher grade B
Graduate entry requirements	• 2:1 or higher in any discipline (biology and chemistry minimum to AS-level)
Make-up of interview panel	• Two people: one health professional and one lay person, of whom one male, one female
Months in which interviews are held	• November, December, February
Proportion of overseas students	• 0%
Proportion of mature students	• 20%
Proportion of graduate students	• To be confirmed
Faculty's view of students taking a gap year	• Positive
Proportion of students taking intercalated degrees	• New school, no information at present
Possibility of direct entrance to clinical phase	• No
Fees for overseas students	• N/A
Fees for graduates	• See Chapter 6
Ability to transfer to other medical schools	• New school, no information at present
Assistance for elective funding	• Available
Assistance for travel to attachments	• Contact medical school directly for advice
Access and hardship funds	• Available. Pick up a leaflet at the student services reception to apply for hardship funds
Weekly rent	• £40–£60 (private)
Pint of lager	• £2
Cinema	• £2 upward
Nightclub	• £3 upward

Imperial College London

Key facts	Undergraduate
Course length	6 years
Total number of medical undergraduates	c 2000
Applicants in 2003	2315
Interviews given in 2003	900
Places available in 2003	326
Places available in 2004	326
Open days 2004	17 February
Entrance requirements	ABBA
Mandatory subjects	Biology, chemistry
Male:female ratio	44:56
Is an exam included in the selection process? If yes, what form does this exam take?	No
Qualification gained	BSc, MBBS

Imperial College School of Medicine was the product of a merger between Charing Cross and Westminster and St Mary's Schools of Medicine. The first intake on the new course began in autumn 1998, and by 2004 there will be no students left who started at one of the separate medical schools. Imperial College School of Medicine has created a new identity while maintaining the spirit and traditions of the original schools. Research at both medical schools is well respected and strong. The Sir Alexander Fleming building, at the Imperial College site in South Kensington, is very central and only 200 m from Hyde Park. All first-year halls of residence are close to this site. Imperial is now one of the largest medical schools in the country, and the extracurricular elements such as sport and music are flourishing in their new environment. Which other medical students graduate from the Albert Hall?

Education 🖤

Imperial offers a 6-year course incorporating an intercalated Honours year (BSc) for everyone except appropriately qualified graduates. Non-graduate mature students are expected to undertake the 6 years. It combines the best of the traditional medical courses with more emphasis on communication skills, medical ethics and law, and information technology. There is integrated teaching from year 1, which includes early exposure to general practice on a weekly basis combined with laboratory and clinical skills sessions. In years 1 and 2, teaching is based on a term structure (see prospectus) and, as the course takes advantage of the large number of hospitals in west London, a wide variety of clinical experience is offered over many sites. New courses have been introduced, including a business course and an introduction to graduate medical practice, and the integrated course has now matured and adapted to the comments of the pioneering students. This has made it a well-tailored and enjoyable experience.

Teaching

A mixture of exams and continuous assessment is used to monitor students' progress. Problem-based learning in small groups is a key feature of the teaching at Imperial, but lectures remain the mainstay of teaching. Students are encouraged to use computers and clinical skills laboratories located at all the main campuses. Lectures and ward attachments take place during all parts of the course, but as you progress more time is spent on hospital attachments. Anatomy is taught from year 2 by dissection of cadavers. However, most anatomy teaching uses predissected cadavers guided by an anatomist. These are fun weekly sessions.

Assessments

End-of-year exams form the basis of assessment in the first 3 years, with more regular assessments after most firms as you progress into the clinical years. Retakes are offered after all end-of-year exams if things don't go to plan, and are traditionally held in the September before the following academic year. Vivas (oral examinations) have been phased out at Imperial, welcomed by many students as they were considered rather subjective. As a BSc is a compulsory inclusion to the Imperial course (year 4 or 5) this is assessed at the end of the BSc year in a terminal exam, throughout the year via in-course essays, and finally on a BSc project of your choosing.

Intercalated degrees

A compulsory BSc has been built into the new course which is normally undertaken in years 4 or 5. The BSc is a modular degree programme and there is a wide range of subject choices, for example genetics, psychology, biochemistry, and management (taught at the Imperial College Management School alongside MBA students). Some introductory modules are undertaken in year 3 and can count towards the final BSc. Students are also free to apply to other universities for courses not offered by Imperial College.

Special study modules and electives

There is a 12-week elective in year 6 during which time students are encouraged to explore how medicine is practised abroad. Imperial College offers many grants each year to students undertaking valuable study abroad, which helps ease the cost. An SSM in the final year covers a 3-week block in a topic of your choice. There is a wide range of specialties to choose from, ranging from alternative medicine and sports medicine to radiology.

Erasmus

The college participates and has an extensive network within the European Union's SOCRATES-ERASMUS programme of study abroad exchanges. Currently, all SOCRATES-ERASMUS participants who are assessed as eligible (usually through eligible European nationality), receive a mobility grant courtesy of the European Union. Europe is the main area where students pursue the various types of placement abroad. These cover whole year and shorter placements. The Imperial College Union has an ERASMUS Club which aims to help with and improve your preparation. You can obtain further information from Admissions Tutors. Alternatively, you can contact the International Liaison Office by telephoning +44 (0)20 7594 8044 or emailing exchangestudents@imperial.ac.uk.

Facilities

Library   There are libraries at all sites (including peripheral ones), of which most are open from 9 am until 9 pm on weekdays and also on Saturday mornings. They do hold reference copies of all recommended texts, but loan copies generally disappear quite quickly. All libraries also hold videos of clinical lectures, so that if you miss one or don't understand one, you can always review it at your leisure – you can't always make every 9 am! Centrally given lectures are also "beamed" out to the peripheral hospitals so that you never miss important lectures if you are on an outside placement.

Computers   There is a considerable emphasis on IT in the Imperial course. To sustain this, the number of computer facilities has expanded considerably, and IT training is provided formally in year 1. The Charing Cross campus has recently installed new machines, some with CD writers, and there are computer facilities for Imperial College medical students at all peripheral attachments as well.

Clinical skills   There are clinical skill labs at Charing Cross and St Mary's hospitals and at some peripheral hospitals too. Students are encouraged to use them as part of their training in both timetabled and student-arranged sessions. They are very well equipped and good fun to use. You can practise everything from taking blood to doing a rectal examination on latex dummies. These help you build confidence before doing procedures on real patients.

Welfare

Student support

Students, based at South Kensington in year 1, can feel remote from the medical environment. However, soon after starting at Imperial, each fresher is allocated a "parent" student (of the opposite sex) from the year above. "Parents" are able to help freshers adjust to university and medical school life and help them to ease into the social scene. They can also offer advice and tips about the course, and they may even cook their children the odd dinner! Each student is also allocated a tutor, who should be available for personal and academic problems and advice. However, the reality is that some students may go through 6 years without ever meeting this "parent". Imperial College has counselling and welfare services available to all students.

Accommodation

First-years have a guaranteed place in halls from £50 (triple room) to about £85 per week for a single. Halls vary from 2–30 minutes away from one of the three main hospitals, and no more than 1 hour from all the peripheral sites. Private sector accommodation is expensive if you want to live near to Imperial College in South Kensington (£90–£100+ per week). However, as you will spend the majority of your time from your second year onwards based in the Hammersmith hospitals, most students live in and around Hammersmith where rent is less expensive but still quite high between £85 and £100.

Placements

The school uses a wide range of centres across central and west London for teaching. The main teaching hospitals – Charing Cross (Hammersmith), Chelsea and Westminster (Fulham), and St Mary's (Paddington) – are supplemented by peripheral district general hospitals and teaching hospitals in Middlesex and Surrey. The Sir Alexander Fleming building at the main Imperial College site is used for basic biomedical sciences, which constitutes much of year 1. There are good public transport links between all sites, and a London Transport discount scheme has reduced the travel costs. However, getting home from some of the peripheral hospitals can be difficult so accommodation is generally provided if this is the case.

Students experience a wide range of clinical attachments, starting with a GP practice placement in year 1. Initially many attachments will be near to Imperial College, but, as you proceed into your specialist clinical studies (years 4–6), they may be further afield (outside London).You are generally offered a shortlist of hospitals to choose from.

Location of clinical placement/name of hospital	Distance away from medical school (miles)	Difficulty getting there on public transport*	Accommodation available
Charing Cross	4	+	No
Chelsea	1.5	+	No
Ashford, Kent	17	+++	Yes
Hemel Hempstead	27	+++	Yes
Gloucester	130	+++	Yes

*Ease of accessibility: +, set your alarm clock early; ++, long journey; +++, car is a must

Sports and social 🏆

City life

Nothing written in a small paragraph could do justice to the multitude of activities, events, venues, clubs, and locations that London offers. Suffice to say that, if you went to a different restaurant, cinema, ice rink, museum, or club each day for the 6 years you are here, there would still be more to see! Where else can you see Americans suspended in glass boxes for months and "Spiderman" grind a city to a halt?

University life

The medical school has made a name for itself by incorporating the best of both its parent schools. The central London setting and the wide range of people have assisted this process. Opportunities for non-medical pursuits abound, but the traditional medical student lifestyle is in no danger of disappearing. The medical school's own Students' Union and societies help Imperial medics maintain a separate identity from the rest of Imperial College students. However, medical students are still able to take advantage of Imperial College Union and its teams and clubs. There is a newly refurbished student bar at the Charing Cross campus, which holds regular events (however, no one seems to know how to turn the air conditioning on!). Highlights of the year include the fresher's roadshow, the interyear rugby match, rag week, including the Circle line pub crawl, and the summer ball. There are plenty of medical student events spread through each term organised by either the medical school union or individual clubs and societies.

Sports life

Imperial College medical school teams have grounds at Teddington (previously home to England RFC) and Cobham, and Imperial College has pitches and an astroturf at Gunnersbury. Students can also use one of three Imperial College-owned sports centres. The Imperial medics rugby team (old boys including JPR Williams) has already made a name for itself at a European level, and the school frequently holds many United Hospitals trophies. A substantial financial rugby scholarship is also awarded annually to the fresher who has made the greatest impression at the club. Rowing at Imperial College is world class and training facilities reflect this. Women's sports are well established, with hockey and netball being among the most popular. The men's cricket team pride themselves on their post-match celebrations. Other sports include water polo, mountaineering, surfing, and mixed lacrosse, to name but a few. The variety of sporting choice is paralleled only by the mixture of abilities: from the social players to the semiprofessionals and internationals – all are welcome and encouraged.

Fascinating fact: The triangular teabag was invented at Imperial College!

Great things about Imperial 👍

- The opportunities available here will ensure that you leave with the greatest of experiences.
- State-of-the-art audiovisual system, meaning that, if you are at one site and the lecture is at another, it can be beamed to your site; this reduces the need to travel and hence cost.
- You can choose between the close-knit medical community at the medical school, the larger Imperial College environment, or metropolitan city life.
- A brand new building for biomedical sciences, at the South Kensington Imperial College site, as well as Chelsea and Westminster Hospital (known as the "Hilton Hospital") means salubrious surroundings.
- Large city with a huge range of cultural activities – anything you want can be found.

Bad things about Imperial 👎

- 2003 intake was so large there is no lecture theatre big enough to hold the whole year.
- Travel between sites adds to the expense of studying and can be stressful.
- Split teaching at different sites can divide the year group up.
- Imperial College is sometimes pictured as boring and academic. But remember that's NOT the medics!
- Expensive, polluted, overpopulated, time-consuming, dirty old London.

Further information

School of Medicine
Imperial College
London SW7 2AZ
Tel: 020 7594 8056
Fax: 020 7594 8004
Email: admitmed@ic.ac.uk
Web: http://www.med.ic.uk

Additional application information

Average A-level requirements	• ABB in three A-levels and grade A in AS-level
Average Scottish Higher requirements	• Not acceptable unless offered in conjunction with A-levels or Advanced Highers. Contact admissions office for advice on subjects
Graduate entry requirements	• 2:1 in any discipline, 3 A-levels at grade C (including chemistry and biology)
Make-up of interview panel	• Chair, clinician, academic, clinical student
Months in which interviews are held	• November–April
Proportion of overseas students	• 7%
Proportion of mature students	• 2.5%
Proportion of graduate students	• c 7%
Faculty's view of students taking a gap year	• Encouraged provided it is used constructively
Proportion of students taking intercalated degrees	• Compulsory (graduates of disciplines related to medicine permitted to apply for exemption)
Possibility of direct entrance to clinical phase	• Oxbridge only
Fees for overseas students	• Over £100 000
Fees for graduates	• £1125
Ability to transfer to other medical schools	• Contact admissions for further information
Assistance for elective funding	• Based on contribution to medical school and/or hardship reasons
Assistance for travel to attachments	• None available
Access and hardship funds	• Several funds are available to all students
Weekly rent	• £41 (halls-triple room)–£120 (private)
Pint of lager	• £2.70
Cinema	• £7.00
Nightclub	• Free–£20

Leeds

Key facts	Undergraduate
Course length	5 years
Total number of medical undergraduates	1100
Applicants in 2003	2105
Interviews given in 2003	770
Places available in 2003	223
Places available in 2004	238
Open days 2004	June and September
Entrance requirements	AAB
Mandatory subjects	Chemistry
Male:female ratio	37:63
Is an exam included in the selection process? If yes, what form does this exam take?	No
Qualification gained	MBChB

The course at Leeds has undergone several changes recently and there is now a new integrated curriculum: out with the old subject-based teaching of anatomy, biochemistry, physiology, and similar, and in with a module-based integrated course. There is some clinically oriented teaching from year 1, and hospital-based teaching starts towards the end of year 2. The medical school staff have been receptive to any balanced criticisms and suggestions, and this has generated a student-friendly atmosphere. A dedicated Medical Students' Representative Committee (MSRC) has ensured that the course has undergone the necessary changes to iron out faults in the curriculum and the course is proving increasingly popular with new entrants. The medical school attracts a tremendous mix of applicants from up and down the country, as well as overseas and mature students, and the MEDSOC works hard to cater for everyone and ensure that all students have a great time. Medics can sometimes feel a little separated from the rest of the student population, but most get a chance to mix in halls of residence and through sports clubs.

Education

The course is systems-based and incorporates clinical experience from year 1. Modules include personal and professional development, biomedical sciences I & II, transport systems of the body, nutrition and energy, control and movement, life cycle, medical and surgical specialities, psychiatry, primary care, public health, and obstetrics and gynaecology. In addition, a great deal of importance is placed on special study components.

Teaching

Teaching is integrated, with a mix of problem-solving exercises, small group teaching, and lectures. The use of computer-based learning is increasing rapidly; with experiments, tutorials, and practice test questions being placed on the intranet. Anatomy is still taught using dissection of human cadavers in years 1–3. Ward teaching begins in year 2 and is split between Leeds General Infirmary, St James' Hospital, and Bradford Royal Infirmary.

Assessment

Assessments include integrated examinations consisting of multiple-choice questions and extended multiple questions (matching the right answer to the right question) with a chance to do a formative exam to help students see how much they need to revise! Special study components count towards a major part of the assessment and objective structured clinical examinations occur in years 3, 4, and 5.

Intercalated degrees

At Leeds, students have a choice whether or not they want to do an extra year to gain a BSc. This can be taken after the years 2, 3, and 4. The number of places available for intercalating has recently been increased and there is a range of scholarships on offer.

Special study modules and electives

Special study modules, referred to as SSCs at Leeds, occur throughout the course. These include three short projects in year 1, two in both years 2 and 3, three in year 4, and four in year 5. There is a wide variety of subjects on offer and in addition, individuals have the opportunity of creating their own. As well as medical SSCs, students also have the option of studying languages, working with the police and taking part in scientific and community projects.

A 10-week elective is timetabled at the beginning of year 5 – the first week in August to the first week in October. Many students travel overseas for this, and recent destinations have included Canada, Australia, Africa, and Barbados.

Erasmus

Currently medical students at Leeds are not part of the Erasmus scheme. However, they do have the opportunity to study abroad for their elective.

Facilities

Library   The medical school has its own well-stocked library shared with dentists and nurses. It is open until 9 pm Monday to Thursday (12 pm near exams), 7 pm on Friday and 5 pm on Saturday. Medical students also have access to the other two libraries in the university.

Computers   There is very good provision of modern computers throughout Leeds University and at St James' Hospital (Jimmy's). There is an IT course at the beginning of year 1 to help those who need to update or expand their computer literacy.

Clinical skills   There are clinical skills laboratories at St James' Hospital, Leeds General Infirmary (LGI), and Bradford Royal Infirmary.

Welfare

Student support

There is a wide level of support at Leeds ranging from the MUMS (where first years are paired with a "parent" from a later year), to a personal tutor scheme and the counselling services available in the university. The MUMS scheme has been running for a number of years and enables students from different years to interact with first-years to provide support and encouragement. The personal tutor scheme matches every student with a doctor who is a point of contact for personal and academic issues. In addition, the first and second year students have the opportunity to meet with the academic deans to discuss their progress and highlight any fears or anxieties they may have. Finally, the Students Union and the university have excellent counselling services.

Accommodation

All first-years can live in university accommodation; either halls or flats. These can be pricey, but standards are generally good and it can be an excellent way to meet non-medics. In year 2 most move out to back-to-back houses in Leeds. Rents start at about £45 per week, but most pay a little more. Insurance is costly, and burglary can be a problem. Although locals can sometimes be a little antistudent, this is not generally a problem as the majority of students all live so close to one another. There is help in finding accommodation available from the university through the Unipol scheme.

Placements

The medical school is attached to the Leeds General Infirmary (one of the main teaching hospitals). The city centre is a 10-minute walk from the school, and free shuttle buses run from the LGI to

Location of clinical placement/name of hospital	Distance away from medical school (miles)	Difficulty getting there on public transport*	Accommodation available
Leeds General Infirmary	0	+	No
Bradford Royal Infirmary	15	+++	No
Chapel Allerton Hospital	3.5	+	No
Cookridge Hospital	5.4	+	No
Airdale General Hospital	20.7	+++	Yes

*Ease of accessibility: +, set your alarm clock early; ++, long journey; +++, car is a must

St James' and to the other hospitals that students may need to attend. Facilities in the teaching hospitals are generally of a high standard. The three main teaching hospitals are Jimmy's, LGI, and BRI. Many district general hospitals are used, including York, Harrogate, Ilkley, Halifax, Scunthorpe, Otley, Hull, Huddersfield, and Wakefield. A few third-year students spend a term in the Yorkshire Dales. In years 4 and 5, attachments can be even further afield. All accommodation and transport is provided for residential attachments. Travel costs are variable and are to a certain degree supported by the university, although students are expected to carry the bulk of the cost. Leeds medical school's district hospitals incorporate the majority of West and North Yorkshire, with Sheffield medical school serving South Yorkshire. It depends where you live in Leeds, but the furthest you may have to travel is Hull (about 60 miles), which can take well over an hour in rush-hour traffic.

Sports and social 🏆

City life

Leeds is the fastest-growing city in the UK outside London. The main city centre has all the shopping and nightlife that your bank account can take, within a 10–15-minute walk from main campus. Leeds also has a theatre, many museums, and galleries, which cater for the culture vultures. Sport is big in Leeds, especially football, cricket, and rugby league.

"Possibly the shopping capital of the north!" The city centre boasts the first Harvey Nichols outside London, and with the many other shops, there is everything anyone could want. The Yorkshire Dales are a short bus journey away and a fantastic place to walk and get away from the hustle and bustle of life in Leeds. There are good road links and Leeds is on the Intercity rail network.

University life

The Union has four bars, including the biggest in Europe (allegedly). MedSoc is probably the most active society of the Union and organises endless events, including two annual balls, pub-crawls, ice-skating, quizzes, ballet trips, and lots of general drinking nights – something for everyone. The university also has a wide range of clubs and societies.

Sports life

Medics' rugby, football, hockey, netball, cricket, and racket games are all supported by the MSRC. The university has a large sports centre, loads of gym equipment, aerobics classes, yoga, kickboxing, etc. The main university runs many sports teams as well.

Fascinating fact: You can fit a mini into the lifts in the medical school.

Great things about Leeds 👍

- The friendliness among medics between different years.
- The Leeds nightlife means that there is always something for everyone to do.
- Very active medical student committees organise everything from balls to sports events.
- Proximity to the Dales – a city in the country!
- Leeds is a city on the up and there is a definite buzz about the centre (and fantastic shopping), with an impressive new Millennium Square.

Bad things about Leeds 👎

- There are so many distractions from studying.
- Medics always seem to have exams and assessments when the rest of the university doesn't, and vice versa.
- Increased use of computers can lead to problems of access.
- Traffic, particularly at rush-hour, and many road works are choking the city centre.
- Everywhere in Leeds is hilly!

Further information

Admissions Office
School of Medicine
University of Leeds
Leeds LS2 9JT
Tel: 0113 233 4362
Fax: 0113 233 4375
Email: prospectus@leeds.ac.uk
Web: http://www.leeds.ac.uk

Additional application information

Average A-level requirements	• AAB at A-level or AB (plus AA at AS Level). A-level chemistry required. General studies not accepted
Average Scottish Higher requirements	• AAAAB at Highers with BB at Advanced Higher level (chemistry required)
Graduate entry requirements	• 2:1 (in a science based degree)
Make-up of interview panel	• Two staff members (from medical school academic staff, NHS Consultants, and GPs) plus one medical student
Months in which interviews are held	• December, January, February, March
Proportion of overseas students	• 6%
Proportion of mature students	• 5%
Proportion of graduate students	• 5%
Faculty's view of students taking a gap year	• Encouraged for those wishing to gain work experience, voluntary work or travel
Proportion of students taking intercalated degrees	• 40%
Possibility of direct entrance to clinical phase	• There is now an integrated curriculum
Fees for overseas students	• £10 307 pa (preclinical) £19 367 pa (clinical)
Fees for graduates	• £1125
Ability to transfer to other medical schools	• This option is not encouraged due to the integration of the course
Assistance for elective funding	• Yes, although applications with projects are more successful than those for clinical attachments
Assistance for travel to attachments	• No – responsibility of LEA/ELB/SAAS
Access and hardship funds	• Yes
Weekly rent	• Halls £50–95; private £50–75
Pint of lager	• £1.30 union; £2.50 city centre
Cinema	• £3–5
Nightclub	• £3–6

Leicester

Key facts	Undergraduate	Graduate
Course length	5 years	4 years
Total number of medical undergraduates	1000	64
Applicants in 2003	1500	400
Interviews given in 2003	800	200
Places available in 2003	175	64
Places available in 2004	175	64
Open days 2004	28 April	
Entrance requirements	AAA	2:1 minimum
Mandatory subjects	Chemistry and biology	Health sciences
Male:female ratio	60:40	20:68
Is an exam included in the selection process? If yes, what form does this exam take?	No	No
Qualification gained	MBChB	MBChB

Leicester is a young medical school whose first students graduated in 1980. It is a friendly place, with the teaching for Phase I being on the university campus in the Maurice Shock Building (MSB), which is next to Victoria Park about 10–15 minutes' walk from the city centre. Most of the main halls are further out in one of the nicer areas of Leicester and they have beautiful gardens. The later phases of the course are based mainly at the Clinical Sciences Building (CSB). This is part of Leicester Royal Infirmary and is close to the city centre. The Union provides many a good night out, and there is also a wide range of nights out and other events organised by LUSUMA (Leicester's Medical Student Society), including balls, outings, and skiing trips.

In 2003, the 5-year course in Leicester was joined by a new 4-year course in medicine for health science graduates. The 4-year accelerated course is the second of the Leicester–Warwick Medical Schools programmes to offer graduates a specialised programme of study.

Approximately 10% of students on the 5-year course are mature students and there is a good representation of international students from a variety of countries.

Education

In common with most other medical schools, Leicester has largely done away with the traditional preclinical/clinical divide. The 5-year course is now separated into two phases, each lasting 2.5 years. Phase I is taught in the MSB and is structured around tutorials and lectures. There is, however, an introduction to clinical skills and you are let loose on wards in November of year 2. Anatomy is taught using dissection and prosections. Phase II is mainly clinical, with ward teaching in different specialties, and includes an elective period in March of year 4. Progression between the two phases is subject to passing examinations. Phase I lasts 1.5 years for the 4-year course and students then join with the fifth-year students for Phase II.

In written examinations, extra time is given to those with specific educational needs such as dyslexia.

Under current arrangements, the PRHO matching scheme launches in September with students informed of allocation in December (further information available at www.lnrdeanery.nhs.uk).

Teaching

For Phase I teaching, students are placed in a group of eight for tutorial work and will remain with this group throughout the phase. Four tutorial groups share a room and tutor. Phase II teaching is on the wards, but it is backed by some lectures in the form of an academic half-day each week. Students are placed with a clinical partner of choice and attendance is registered and contributes to passing each clinical attachment. There are 13 x 8-week blocks, which rotate through disciplines and include an elective. For each block, the pair of clinical students is attached to two consultant teams of different specialities.

Assessment

Module examinations are mainly written short-answer questions or assessed essays. There is a 15-station OSCPE (Objective Structured Clinical and Practical Exam) examination at the end of semester two. Assessment in Phase II includes patient portfolios (case studies) and clinical skills (histories and examinations). Finals have a clinical component and written examinations.

Intercalated degrees

Any student wishing to do an Honours year is encouraged to do so. Honours degrees can be science-based or clinical and there is a wide range of subjects to choose from. Students have the option of intercalating after either years 2 or 3 of study assuming that their academic performance is good enough.

Special study modules and electives

All students have a 2-month elective module, which can be carried out in the UK or abroad and takes place during March of year 4.

Two special study modules (SSM) are taken in Phase I, and one in Phase II. It is compulsory to study one science SSM, although other subjects such as languages are available for the second.

Erasmus

Leicester has recently entered the MedSIN/IFMSA exchange programme organised by the MedSIN National Officer for Professional Exchanges. This allows clinical students to directly switch places with a foreign student for a 4-week period. Furthermore, there is an opportunity in year 3 to spend 10 weeks on a short Erasmus exchange to Germany (Saarland), Spain (Grenada), and in French-speaking Switzerland. Some knowledge of the native language is advisable when you apply for Erasmus programmes. The disadvantage is that upon returning from exchanges in December, students must sit the Phase I examination in January. However, staff are supportive if asked for help with revision.

Facilities

Library   The main university library is on campus, near to the MSB, and is open until midnight during the week. There are also medical libraries at the three main teaching hospitals. The CSB library at the Leicester Royal Infirmary is the largest of these and opens 24 hours, making it popular around examination times! It is staffed between 9 am and 10 pm on weekdays. The staffed hours are shorter on Saturday (9 am–6 pm) and Sunday (2 pm–9 pm).

Computers   There are computer facilities for all university students on the main campus in the main library, Charles Wilson and Kenneth Edward buildings. The MSB has a computer room for medical students, which has recently been refitted with new computers. There are also PCs available at the clinical sciences libraries at all three University Hospitals of Leicester sites. Course work (case studies and essays) must be word-processed. The medical school is gradually introducing online assessments in some modules.

Clinical skills   Clinical skills at Leicester begin during year 1 of study. This initially takes the form of interviewing "simulated patients" as well as practising physical examination skills on volunteers. These skills are examined at the end of year 1 in the form of OSCPEs. This progresses in year 2 to clinical placements one morning per week in one of the Leicester hospitals, where the skills learnt in year 1 are revised and put into practice.

Welfare

Student support

Each tutor group is allocated a personal tutor and they are nominated faculty members with a pastoral role. Overall, the faculty staff at the MSB are very approachable and supportive. Each hospital has a student facilitator to deal with queries and problems and there is always a member of staff available (24 hours) if there are any major problems or emergencies. Leicester University has a self-referral counselling service and the university Nightline offers support and guidance to students (including telephone numbers for taxis and late night food delivery!). Most areas of the medical school and university have standard disabled access facilities, such as ramps and lifts. Anyone with specific requirements would be advised to check with the university.

Accommodation

University accommodation is available throughout the degree, and some medical students stay in university accommodation beyond year 1. In year 1 it is popular – and advisable – to live in catered halls, as there are loads of activities and great end-of-term balls and parties. Stamford has one of the best summer balls of all the university halls. Privately rented accommodation is inexpensive but variable in quality. It is best to shop around in advance for a good deal. A Union-run accommodation office can help you find places and there are many notices on the medical school notice boards for house shares.

Placements

Phase I is based on the university campus in the MSB, and Phase II is based in the CSB/Robert Kilpatrick Building at the Leicester Royal Infirmary (LRI). The LRI is only a 10-minute walk from the MSB, and everything is in reasonable proximity. Teaching also takes place at the Leicester General and Glenfield General Hospitals, which are a short bus ride or, for the energetic, a cycle ride away. There is no student parking available at either the university or the LRI, but there is plenty of free parking at either Glenfield or the General. The medical school is currently undergoing an investment programme that will see a new multidisciplinary medical sciences teaching building being built at the Leicester General Hospital site. In addition, district general hospitals are used in Kettering, Grantham, Northampton, Warwick, Coventry, Nuneaton, Boston, Lincoln, Burton-on-Trent, and Peterborough, where free accommodation is provided. GP attachments are in Leicester and the surrounding area, with the furthest away being in Rugby.

Location of clinical placement/name of hospital	Distance away from medical school (miles)	Difficulty getting there on public transport*	Accommodation available
Leicester Royal Infirmary	0.5	+	No
Leicester General Hospital	2.5	+	No
Peterborough District Hospital	40	+++	Yes
Pilgrim Hospital, Boston	65	+++	Yes
Nuneaton	25	+++	Yes

*Ease of accessibility: +, set your alarm clock early; ++, long journey; +++, car is a must

Sports and social 🏆

City life

The city centre is about a 45-minute walk from halls, or 10–15 minutes from the university campus. There is a regular bus service between halls, the town centre, and the university during term time and a student bus pass available, which gives discounted travel. A good range of cinemas, theatres, pubs, clubs, bars, and shops manages to reflect the city's diverse ethnicity. There are plenty of restaurants, and curry lovers in particular have a wide choice. There are popular clubs in town and late bars to suit all tastes. Many top bands come to Leicester on tour visiting De Montfort Hall and De Montfort University. The "Charlotte" is also a renowned venue for smaller events and is frequented by several popular bands. Leicester has all the facilities of a city as well as some of the homeliness and friendliness of a smaller town.

The city is reasonably small, but has recently been redeveloped and has all the shops you could want. If you have your own transport, the Leicestershire countryside is attractive and makes a pleasant escape from the city. There is Premiership football and world-class rugby on the doorstep.

University life

At the Students' Union there are club nights every Wednesday, Thursday, Friday, and some Saturdays. There are also university events at local clubs – such as the exotically named Zanzibar every week. The Redfearn bar is open all day weekdays and food is available – it proves a popular place to relax after lectures or exams. "Elements", found in the Union building, is open from 10 am serving coffees and snacks. LUSUMA arrange social events every term, such as Halloween parties, a medic's revue, a "Stars in their Eyes" show, and an annual medics ball. There is a large variety of university societies to choose from: some are a bit mad, but if you want to join a society, you will be spoilt for choice and it is a great way to meet students from other courses. The university provides safe transport for all students with its night minibuses, which take students from the campus to anywhere within the city limits. The buses run from approximately 6 pm in the winter (7 pm in summer) until the union closes at 2 am. You can buy a minibus card, which gets you a "free ride", or each journey currently costs £1.

Sports life

Medical students have the opportunity to join university sporting teams (of which there are many) as well as the wide range of medic sporting teams available. Thanks to team captains and the sporting secretaries, there have been vast improvements in recent years in the organisation of the teams. Many teams receive sponsorship from local businesses. There are often sports days at home and away against other medical schools. The university has sports fields at Stoughton Road, two sports halls, two gyms, where there are circuits and aerobic classes, and an athletics track. There are plenty of swimming pools in town, or one near the university halls in Oadby. The medical school adheres (during Phase I) to the non-scheduling of afternoon lessons on Wednesdays when matches take place.

Fascinating fact: Leicester was the first medical school to introduce the integrated style of curriculum (in response to the GMC's *Tomorrow's Doctors*).

Great things about Leicester

- Students and staff are friendly and welcoming.
- There are wide-ranging activities available for all organised by LUSUMA, the Union, and other societies.
- Great improvement in Leicester's nightlife in recent years, with many new bars, clubs, and restaurants for varying tastes.
- Leicester was ranked number 1 in the "Guardian" teaching league tables in 2003.
- Clear module objectives to assist with self directed learning.

Bad things about Leicester

- The location of placements can present you with travel problems.
- Lack of temperature control in lecture theatres.
- Phase II students are spread about the region.
- Not near the sea. In fact, Leicester is about as far from it as you can be.
- No student car parking at the university and Leicester Royal Infirmary.

Further information

Dr Kevin West
Maurice Shock Medical Sciences Building
Leicester University
University Road
Leicester LE1 7RH
Tel: 0116 252 2969/2985
Fax: 0116 252 3013
Email: med-admis@le.ac.uk
Web: http://www.lwms.ac.uk

Additional application information

Average A-level requirements	• AAA, including chemistry and biology
Average Scottish Higher requirements	• AAAAA, including chemistry and biology
Graduate entry requirements	• 2:1 in a health sciences degree
Make-up of interview panel	• One academic, one final year student
Months in which interviews are held	• November–March
Proportion of overseas students	• 8%
Proportion of mature students	• 10%
Proportion of graduate students	• 10%
Faculty's view of students taking a gap year	• Supported
Proportion of students taking intercalated degrees	• 10%
Possibility of direct entrance to clinical phase	• No
Fees for overseas students	• £9990
Fees for graduates	• £1125
Ability to transfer to other medical schools	• Acceptable if students are able to find another medical school which will take them
Assistance for elective funding	• Interest free loan available for travel
Assistance for travel to attachments	• None – responsibility of LEA/ELB/SAAS
Access and hardship funds	• Applications via welfare office
Weekly rent	• £40–£45 (private accommodation)
Pint of lager	• £1.20 in hall bars; £2.20 in the city
Cinema	• £3.60
Nightclub	• Free–£5

Liverpool

Key facts	Undergraduate	Graduate
Course length	5 years	4 years
Total number of medical undergraduates	1265	32
Applicants in 2003	1672	285
Interviews given in 2003	1000	92
Places available in 2003	281	32
Places available in 2004	281	32
Open days 2004	28 April and 13 October	
Entrance requirements	AAB	2:1 degree and BCC
Mandatory subjects	Biology and chemistry	Biomedical or health sciences degree
Male:female ratio	40:60	20:80
Is an exam included in the selection process? If yes, what form does this exam take?	No	No
Qualification gained	MBChB	MBChB

In 1996 Liverpool Medical School introduced a brand new curriculum, in accordance with GMC guidelines. So far it is proving to be a success and August 2001 saw the first PBL (problem-based learning) students to qualify at Liverpool starting on wards as PRHOs. Liverpool Medical School is growing in size, with over 1200 undergraduates, but a strong Medical Students' Society ensures that there is always a friendly face around. Many new buildings and developments are being constructed, and now Liverpool has been awarded the mantle of 2008 City of Culture, it is only going to attract more investment. Liverpool certainly promises to be a special city in the years to come.

Education

Studies follow the human lifecycle, from conception and birth through adulthood and into old age. Since the introduction of the new PBL course, subjects are no longer taught in lecture theatres day in, day out: instead, different areas of medicine are presented to students as problems. Students discuss the issues and formulate learning objectives in small groups with tutor guidance. They then go away and research the information for themselves. From the beginning of year 2 an increasing proportion of time is spent on hospital and community attachments.

Teaching

The new course contains little in the way of formal teaching. The few plenaries (lectures) that are given are designed to provide an overview only of each problem in a brand spanking new lecture theatre (plenary theatre). It is then up to the student to find out further details from the other resources available. Alongside library work, students have formal training in clinical and communication skills. Anatomy is demonstrated using models and prosections in a recently refurbished and improved multimillion pound Human Anatomy Resource Centre, and information technology has an ever-increasing role, with various computer-based learning packages available.

The new 4-year course promises to provide an excellent accelerated course for graduates that encompasses all the aspects of the 5-year course in a condensed form: the first 2 years of the extended course are merged into year 1. Students are pushed hard and the work schedule is not for the faint-hearted but the rewards are proportional to the work you put in.

Assessment

Assessment is continuous, designed so that everything you learn (including practical skills acquired) will be recognised and recorded. Formal exams now occur at the end of every year and at the moment there are no exams in the final year! The final year is spent in five 8-week rotations consisting of two options plus general practice, emergency medicine, and ward shadowing designed to prepare students for the realities of the house job.

Intercalated degrees

It is possible to study for an intercalated degree at the end of year 4. Subjects available include anatomy, biochemistry, cell biology, pharmacology, physiology, psychology, and healthcare ethics. Students at Liverpool can study at BSc, BA, or Master's level, depending on the degree course taken. Some students study for an intercalated degree at another university and then return to complete the medical course at Liverpool. Limited funding is available to some students wishing to study for an intercalated year.

Special study modules and electives

SSM: There are four special study modules each lasting 4 weeks and spread through the first 4 years. They cover a variety of topics. An additional one (the 5th) allows a more in depth study of a topic lasting one day a week for two-thirds of the year. Topics from any specialty can be chosen, and an essay must be completed for each module with some students having their findings published. In addition, in the final year there are the two SAMPs – selective in advanced medical practice. These are 8-week placements spent in a specialty chosen by the student.

Elective: The elective takes place at the end of year 3 from June to the start of September. This is widely regarded as the most exciting part of most medical courses. Applications for placements are aided by a wide network of contacts all over the world.

Erasmus

Two exchange schemes – Socrates and Erasmus – allow students to study at a participating European medical school for a period of 16 weeks during the final year. Current exchanges are set up with schools in France, Germany, Holland, and Sweden. The scheme has recently been expanded to include Eastern European countries.

Facilities

Library   A short-loan system operates for the books most in demand. The library is open until 9.30 pm most weekdays. Opening hours are more restricted at weekends and outside the main university terms, which differ from the medical school terms. All hospitals have their own libraries, and borrowing arrangements for students vary. The books stocked are directly influenced by the demands of the students so the latest books are always available, complemented by an array of electronic journals.

Computers   The university and hospitals have 24-hour computer facilities available for students, with free use of email and the internet.

Clinical skills   One of the real highlights of the new course has been the introduction of the clinical skills laboratory, where students are able to master a whole range of practical doctoring skills, from taking blood and suturing wounds to giving advanced CPR. There are weekly classes in year 1, with a clinical skills exam at the end. Most students agree it is the best part of the week.

Welfare

Student support

Students generally mix well and there are good relations within and between year groups. There is a long-standing mentoring system set up by the LMSS (Liverpool Medical Students Society), so that each first-year student is paired with a second- or third-year student. In recent years Liverpool has enjoyed a very constructive and student-friendly atmosphere within the faculty. In addition to facilities provided by LMSS, the Students' Union has the standard welfare and counselling services.

Accommodation

Most people only live in university accommodation for their first year. This is a good opportunity to meet other students from outside the medical school, but university accommodation is more expensive than renting privately. There is a wide variation in the standard of private accommodation,

Location of clinical placement/name of hospital	Distance away from medical school (miles)	Difficulty getting there on public transport*	Accommodation available
Royal Liverpool Hospital	0	+	No
Arrowe Park	6	++/+++	No
Chester	25	+++	No
Lancaster	70	+++	Yes
Barrow	100	+++	Yes

*Ease of accessibility: +, set your alarm clock early; ++, long journey; +++, car is a must

but there is plenty of choice. The university has no input into regulating the private sector, but the accommodation office can offer advice.

Placements

Liverpool University was the original redbrick university. The campus dominates a large area adjacent to the city centre and between the two cathedrals. The University Hospital is right next to the university campus, and the medical school is well placed near to all the main university and hospital departments.

The medical school is part of a large teaching hospital, the Royal Liverpool University Hospital. Also within the city centre is the Liverpool Women's Hospital, which has 200+ beds. Liverpool has its share of regional specialist centres, including Broadgreen Cardiothoracic Centre, and Alder Hey Children's Hospital in the suburbs. University Hospital Aintree is the other main teaching hospital used by second- and third-year students and is located about 6 miles from the university.

In year 1 all teaching is done in the university. From year 2 onwards, more time is spent on placements. For example, on a typical 2-week module in year 2, one day is spent in a local GP practice and two days are spent either in a relevant community attachment or at one of the hospitals. Placements are mainly within or near to Liverpool (Wirral, Southport, Warrington, Halton, etc.), but some are further away, such as Lancaster, Barrow, Rhyl, and Chester. In year 4 you can be placed at Morcombe Bay Trust for the whole year. The teaching is excellent and travelling once there is at a minimum, but it's a fair old hike if you want to come back for someone's birthday!

Sports and social ♆

City life

Liverpool offers an excellent welcome to students. It is a proud yet warm city, with its world-famous accent, sense of humour, two cathedrals, football teams, and maritime history. It was once the biggest port in the British Empire. Having fallen on hard times in the 1970s and 1980s, Liverpool is now very much on the up and investment in the city has never been higher! Many students, from all courses, stay in the area after graduation. The medical school and the student residential areas are well placed for all the attractions, and are adjacent to the many surprisingly beautiful parks within the city. Like many other cities there is crime about, but a commonsense approach will ensure that the good times aren't spoilt. Police statistics show that Liverpool is, in fact, one of the safest cities in the UK.

Liverpool has an excellent social side – every food taste catered for, excellent pubs, several cinemas, sports complexes, and nightclubs of all hues, from 70s clubs upwards. It is also the home of three football teams – Liverpool, Tranmere Rovers, and Everton. The world's most famous annual horse race, the Grand National at Aintree, is not too far away. It's also the birthplace of the little known band "The Beatles". The city is only a short distance from Manchester, North Wales, Chester, and the Lake Diotriot.

University life

LMSS is a major plus for studying medicine in Liverpool. It covers all aspects of medical student life from interaction with the faculty to weekly meetings with guest speakers. There are regular balls, dinners, and social parties, as well as the medics' own orchestra, choir, sports teams, play, and Christmas revue. The university also offers a wide range of different societies. LMSS has its own website at http://www.LMSS.org. There is also a very active and expanding branch of MedSIN.

Sports life

The Medical Society has football, rugby, hockey, netball, basketball, squash, badminton, and cricket teams. Recent additions to the sports teams include Chinese martial arts and a celebrated tiddlywinks team! The university has all these and more! There are plenty of facilities.

Fascinating fact: Liverpool has the oldest active medical society in England.

Great things about Liverpool

- The PBL course is self-directed and self-motivated, and allows you to adapt your learning to your pace.
- Students have a real say in the course at Liverpool, and course organisers are receptive to their suggestions.
- The course prepares students to work effectively as PRHOs through early patient contact and clinical skills training.
- A diverse syllabus allows all aspects of medicine and those affected by illness to be appreciated.
- The LMSS provides a strong backbone to all activities in Liverpool Medical School, from academic issues to social and welfare issues.

Bad things about Liverpool

- The necessary approach to course work at Liverpool can be very different from A-level studies: PBL is not for people who want to be spoon-fed in lectures.
- Hospital placements can be some distance from Liverpool, and travelling by public transport can be time consuming and expensive.
- University facilities are available during university term dates only. Outside these "normal term times", facilities such as the library are operated on restricted "vacation hours", although this is improving.
- The social life within the medical school can be so good that sometimes it is difficult to get to know students from other courses!
- The weather – it can be cold and wet particularly in the winter!

Further information

Admissions Administrator
Faculty of Medicine
1st floor Duncan Building
Daulby Street
Liverpool L69 3GA
Tel: 0151 706 4266
Fax: 0151 706 5667
Email: mbchb@liv.ac.uk
Web: http://www.liv.ac.uk

Additional application information

Average A-level requirements	• AAB, A-level biology and chemistry plus one other
Average Scottish Higher requirements	• AAABB Highers, including chemistry, biology, maths, physics, English. Two Advanced Highers including chemistry
Graduate entry requirements	• 2:1 in biomedical or health sciences
Make-up of interview panel	• Two academic or clinical staff
Months in which interviews are held	• November–March
Proportion of overseas students	• 7.5%
Proportion of mature students	• 3%
Proportion of graduate students	• 13%
Faculty's view of students taking a gap year	• Acceptable (except for the graduate course)
Proportion of students taking intercalated degrees	• 10%
Possibility of direct entrance to clinical phase	• No
Fees for overseas students	• £15 800 pa
Fees for graduates	• £1125
Ability to transfer to other medical schools	• A supportive Faculty will try their best to facilitate any transfer if there are exceptional circumstances. But why would you want to leave Liverpool?!
Assistance for elective funding	• Liverpool Medical Students' Society (LMSS) provides information on available funding
Assistance for travel to attachments	• Only through LEA/ELB/SAAS
Access and hardship funds	• Guild is supportive although remember to keep all those bank statements
Weekly rent	• £30 if you want to be centre of attention with the locals, £40 if you prefer anonymity
Pint of lager	• £1–£1.20 in certain clubs and on campus
Cinema	• £4-ish, a few mainstream choices and an excellent art house cinema, FACT, newly opened
Nightclub	• £1.50–£7. The best has to be the Ras, officially known as the Blue Angel, just never get there sober, or with people you want to impress!

Manchester, Keele, and Preston

		Manchester	Keele
Key facts	Premedical	Undergraduate	Undergraduate
Course length	6 years	5 years	5 years
Total number of medical undergraduates	c 1850		
Applicants in 2003	530	2333	387
Interviews given in 2003	200	1083	229
Places available in 2003	21	341	65
Places available in 2004	21	341	55
Open days 2004	June	21 April	5 May 8 September
Entrance requirements	AAB	AAB	AAB
Mandatory subjects	Non-science	Chemistry	Chemistry
Male:female ratio		44:56	55:45
Is an exam included in the selection process? If yes, what form does this exam take?	No	No	No
Qualification gained	MBChB		

Manchester is home to three universities: the University of Manchester, the Manchester Metropolitan University (MMU), and the University of Manchester Institute of Science and Technology (UMIST). As a result, it boasts a student population of over 50 000. The medical school is part of the University of Manchester and is the second largest in the UK. Medicine has been on the curriculum here since the early 19th century.

The medical campus is situated on Oxford Road, right in the heart of a busy cosmopolitan city, which many now see as the London of the North. In 1994 Manchester was the first UK school to introduce a systems-based problem-based learning curriculum, following the publication of the GMC document *Tomorrow's Doctors*, and so has over 9 years' experience in problem-based learning. Although a preclinical/clinical divide exists, the basic sciences are studied within a clinical framework of patient cases, which are used to direct learning each week.

Manchester is unique in that students are joined in year 3 by an intake of students from St Andrew's. In addition, students may choose to undertake part or all of their training at the new teaching centre of Keele.

Preston, a base hospital of the Lancashire Teaching Hospital NHS Trust, welcomed its first group of year 3 students in September 2003. This new base hospital is a permanent addition to the Manchester Medical Schools and will provide additional medical education posts in the north west.

Manchester

Education

The course is 5 years long, with two preclinical years followed by three clinical ones. The preclinical course is structured around weekly cases that are studied through a mixture of group discussion, practical anatomy and pathology laboratories, computer skills sessions, lecture theatre events, and personal study. The course is organised into four semesters, so that cases relate to the four themes of nutrition and metabolism, cardiorespiratory, abilities and disabilities, and lifecycle. Years 3 and 4 continue the case-based approach in a clinical setting, and the four themes are repeated. Four days per week are spent in one of the five teaching hospitals, and one day per week in a general practice surgery. Year 5 works on a four-block rotation system, whereby an equal number of students will be on an elective, at a teaching hospital, a district general hospital, or in the community at any one time. Because of the high attendance demands on final-year students, free hospital accommodation is provided during attachments, which allows students to shadow house officers and gain practical experience to prepare them for their preregistration house officer jobs.

Teaching

First- and second-year teaching focuses on a weekly case study with supplementary group discussions, lectures, and practical sessions, including microscopy, anatomy, group tutorials, anatomy sessions using cadavers, basic clinical skills, and computational skills. Students work in groups to create weekly learning objectives, which are fulfilled in their own time with the aid of the above resources.

Years 3, 4, and 5 continue to base teaching around a case setting, but students now fulfil learning objectives within a clinical setting. Whereas in year 1 the study objectives in the case of the man with lung cancer involves learning about the pathology of lung cancers from a textbook and pathology specimens, in clinical years students have the opportunity to attend chest clinics and talk to and examine people with the actual disease. In the clinical years, students also receive bedside teaching. In years 3 and 4 there is a maximum of 12 students per firm. Unfortunately, it is not uncommon for sessions to be cancelled, or for sessions to be rescheduled owing to the patient commitments of the medical staff.

Assessment

In years 1 and 2 there are exams at the end of each of the four semesters. They comprise MCQs, two papers on clinical case studies, an exam requiring the interpretation of scientific prose into lay language, an OSSE (objective structured skills examination) and, unusually, a computer skills exam. At the end of each semester, groups are assessed and marked for communication skills and teamwork. For those studying the "European option" there are weekly lessons with homework and exams.

Assessment in years 3 and 4 is twice a year and consists of a Progress Test (Single Best Answer format) and an OSCE. The OSCE sees students rotate through up to 15 x 5-minute stations, where they are presented with various tasks and challenges appropriate to the area that they are being assessed in. For example, students may be asked to interpret laboratory results, examine patients, or deal with ethically challenging situations. In the final year, students take one set of exams in May comprising an OSCE, a patient management paper (PMP), and a final true/false paper.

Intercalated degrees

Intercalated BSc (or MSc) courses are offered at the end of years 2 and 4. There is a wide range of basic bioscience subjects available to study, as well as more unusual subjects such as healthcare ethics and law, and history of medicine, which have proved extremely popular over recent years. Students can choose to intercalate at another institution, but only in a subject not offered at Manchester. Traditionally, students wishing to intercalate would have been expected to have an above average academic record, but the faculty seems to be widening access to any student wishing to intercalate. Some funding is available, and is allocated according to academic merit. Some scholarships are also available from trusts and businesses, depending on the subject studied.

Students may also interrupt the course to complete a PhD.

Special study modules and electives

In years 1 and 2 there is one 4-week special study module (SSM) per year, whereas in years 3 and 4 there are two per year. These modules can be on practically anything, and there is talk of allowing students to do one SSM in a topic unrelated to medicine to encourage the pursuit of other hobbies and interests. Another point to note is that, in the clinical years, one of the SSMs must be in a DGH (district general hospital) and one in the community.

Many students do SSMs at Preston; the Families and Children module has been run at Preston for several years now. Both Chorley and South Ribble DGH have a good record in providing year 5 placements in hospital and community for the Preston course.

At the end of year 4 students undertake a 12-week research project. Students are allocated a supervisor and have the opportunity to pursue a topic that particularly interests them. This period provides an excellent introduction to medical research, and allows students to get to grips with medical statistics. Some students even go on to have their work published.

In the final year there is an elective period, where students are encouraged to go abroad to appreciate medicine in a foreign healthcare setting. The elective officially lasts 8 weeks, but students often piggyback their time onto an adjacent holiday such as Christmas to increase their time away. Students cover costs for electives, so a great deal of organisation and planning is often needed. In addition, a report must be submitted upon returning to Manchester.

Erasmus

Eligible Manchester students are also offered the chance to pursue the "European option". Students who successfully complete this element of the course are awarded a degree which recognises their medical training in the context of a foreign language and healthcare system. Students with good grades in A-level languages can choose to study either French or German in addition to the medicine course. Medical vocabulary is taught from year 1, and 4 months of year 5 are spent at the partner universities of Rennes (France), Saarland (Germany), and Lausanne (Switzerland). The faculty has established good working relationships with these three faculties over a number of years and knows that students receive experience equivalent to that in Manchester. The Medical School is currently considering Spanish as an additional language on the list and it is hoped that this will be available in the very near future.

Facilities

Library   The Medical Faculty library is well equipped with the basic textbooks, but demand is high and it is often busy. It is open 9 am–8 pm during term time, weekdays only. The John Rylands University Library across the road stocks most of the major journals. This library is open from 9 am to 9.30 pm weekdays, and 9 am to 6 pm and 1 pm to 6 pm on Saturday and Sunday, respectively. The opening hours in holiday times are shorter. Hospital libraries vary in size and standard.

Computers   There are excellent computer facilities in the medical school and John Rylands Library, with internet access and email for all. A number of computer-assisted learning programs are available, and computer laboratories in the medical school are open from 9 am to 7 pm. Hospitals also have computer and email facilities.

Clinical skills   More and more emphasis is being placed on the use of skills laboratories, and facilities in the clinical years of the course are being improved. There has been a tremendous influx of money into the skills laboratories over the last 2 years and there is a variety of mannequins for practising such skills as CPR, injections, and blood taking, and video resources on clinical skills are available for viewing.

Welfare

Student support

Faculty staff are extremely approachable and student feedback is consistently encouraged. Student representatives sit on all major faculty committees, and student opinions are frequently sought. In particular, three staff–student liaison meetings are held in each academic year, which give ample opportunity for students to raise issues close to their hearts. Good relationships between students and tutors are fostered through tutorials. Students are also allocated a member of staff who acts as a pastoral tutor, and there are both faculty and Students' Union-based counselling services, which are highly regarded.

Accommodation

University accommodation is guaranteed for first-years, and, although most students choose to move into the private sector after this, some do stay. Halls may be catered or self-catering, and vary in price and standard. There is a lot of private sector accommodation, ranging in price from £37 to £60 per week. Most accommodation is within walking distance of the university, and a short bus ride from the town centre. The last few years have also seen the rise of a number of large commercial accommodation blocks aimed at students, a number of which offer rooms with en-suite facilities, and even onsite gyms and swimming pools!

Placements

In years 3 and 4, four days per week are spent at the base hospital and one day in the community. However, as in most other medical schools, getting to and from placements can be very time consuming without a car. In theory, base hospitals (excluding Keele and Preston) are all within 45 minutes of the university by public transport. However, although having a car can be a general advantage in the clinical years, the public transport network is fast and efficient and can often beat rush-hour traffic! Accommodation at placements is available, but depends on which year you are in. In year 5 accommodation is provided at all sites. However, in years 3 and 4 accommodation is not provided in Preston, Keele, MRI, Hope, or Wythenshawe. All DGH placements for obstetrics and gynaecology, paediatrics, and SSMs offer accommodation.

Location of clinical placement/name of hospital	Distance away from medical school (miles)	Difficulty getting there on public transport*	Accommodation available
Manchester Royal Infirmary	0	+	Yes
Hope Hospital	6	++	Yes
Wythenshawe Hospital	6.5	++	Yes
Preston	39.1	+++	Yes
Keele	45	+++	Yes

*Ease of accessibility: +, set your alarm clock early; ++, long journey; +++, car is a must

Sports and social 🏆

City life

With such a huge student population, Manchester offers an endless choice of where to go and what to do. There is a wide variety of pubs, bars, clubs, stores, theatres, and restaurants, each with a different character, theme, or style. The city is truly multicultural and there is a good mix of home, overseas, mature, and postgraduate students, as well as a vibrant gay and lesbian scene. For those interested in music, Manchester is a fantastic place to study. As well as the local scene, most of the big-name tours include Manchester gigs. However, should all the excitement get too much for you, the Peak District, Pennines, Lake District, and North Wales are not far away for a little peace and tranquillity, along with Liverpool, Leeds, and Sheffield!

University life

The Medical Students' Representative Council (MSRC) is the focus of medical school social life. The 12-strong committee is elected each year by students and organises a number of medics' events throughout the year, including the infamous "pyjama pub crawl" and the annual winter ball. There are also year clubs, which organise trips, parties, and one graduation ball for each year. The medics dramatics society, organises an annual pantomime, and a revue. In addition, the medical school magazine *Mediscope* is published three times a year (on paper and the web) and provides a journalistic forum for the medical student population. Along with faculty events, a huge range of clubs and societies are run from Manchester Students' Union, which is opposite the medical school.

Sports life

Being home to one of the most famous football teams in the world is only the start for Manchester, and, although tickets for United's games can be a little pricey, Manchester City offers cut-price tickets to students for home games. This is probably a blessing in disguise, as the majority of locals living in the student areas are City fans! There is also a discount price for students at Sale Sharks Rugby Club.

Manchester's sports scene has seen huge benefits from the opening of many facilities built to cater for the 2002 Commonwealth Games, which has left a legacy of world-class sporting facilities. Developments include a campus-located Olympic size swimming pool, as well as the creation of the national cycling, squash, and netball centres. The centrepiece of the Commonwealth Games was the 37 000-seat "City of Manchester stadium", which in 2003 became the new home of Manchester City.

Within the medical school, Manchester has a thriving sporting community. There are medics' rugby, hockey, tennis, netball, rowing, and football teams, which actively encourage participation and socialising. The main university also has countless sports clubs, but medics tend to play for the medics' team if one exists in their sport. Most of the medics sports teams have an annual tour which is not to be missed.

Keele

The Universities of Manchester and Keele won funding to provide training and education for undergraduate medics from October 2000 onwards, and also to establish the full 5-year course at Keele from September 2003. Students who wish to study at Keele have the following options:

- 5-year course at Keele
- 5-year course, with years 1 and 2 at Manchester and the final 3 years at Keele
- 6-year course, including a premedical year for students without an appropriate science background at A-level. The premedical year is at Manchester.

An intercalated degree can be incorporated with any of the options. A BSc can be taken at Keele or Manchester. Keele hopes to offer the European option from 2003.

Depending on your choice of the study options listed above, you should apply to either Manchester or Keele (K12). Students undertaking the full 5-year course at Keele will spend years 1 and 2 based primarily on the Keele campus site in the new purpose-built Health Sciences complex.

Keele is a large attractive campus university with restaurants, sports and social facilities, as well as library and academic buildings. The clinical years at Keele will be spent predominantly at the North Staffordshire NHS Hospital Trust, only 3 miles away from Keele. This is a very busy hospital offering the full range of clinical services and is an excellent place to gain clinical experience. In addition, students are guaranteed accommodation on campus for their first year of study.

The structure of the course and the assessments are the same for both Keele and Manchester students. The first students for Keele and North Staffordshire arrived in October 2002, having started in Manchester in October 2000. The local consultants and staff in partner district general hospitals are extremely enthusiastic about teaching medical students.

Until 2007 at the earliest, Keele can only consider applications from home and EU students.

Preston: Lancashire teaching hospitals

Preston forms part of the Lancashire teaching hospitals and was created in August 2002 by the merger of two well-established hospitals. Royal Preston Hospital has a long history and is now a modern building with good transport access. Chorley and South Ribble DGH was extensively rebuilt and enlarged in 1994. Both hospitals have an excellent record in providing placements for Manchester students.

Since September 2003, 30 places per annum have been available for Manchester students to study at the Lancashire teaching hospitals; from 2007 this will increase up to 80 places.

There is a modern education unit at the Chorley site and a new education and training unit under construction at Preston to provide state-of-the-art facilities for learning and teaching. Both centres will have excellent library and IT resources in addition to a well-provided clinical skills unit.

Student accommodation is available within a reasonable distance from the main base hospital at Preston. Access to Manchester is reasonable, journeys are 30–40 minutes by car. Trains are frequent and provide access to central Manchester in 30–40 minutes. Blackpool, Preston, and Wigan have an active nightlife, and Preston has a large student population linked to the University of Central Lancashire.

Fascinating fact: Manchester's first female medical student graduated in 1904.

Great things about Manchester

- Enthusiasm for medicine is maintained by a course that emphasises clinical problems from day 1.
- The faculty staff are very approachable and open to change. There are plenty of opportunities to give feedback on both course and staff.
- The social life is excellent. There are loads of events organised by the MSRC (Medical Students' Representative Council), and there is generally lots going on at reasonable prices.
- The sheer size of the multifaculty universities in Manchester, and the 2002 Commonwealth Games, have ensured top-level academic and sporting facilities.
- In year 3 a load of new people arrive from St Andrew's, which spices things up a bit!

Bad things about Manchester

- Adjusting to self-directed learning can be difficult for some students who are used to being spoon-fed, although this is becoming the case at all UK schools with new courses.
- Differing interpretations of self-directed learning can often mean students perceive a lack of teaching.
- Some hospital placements are quite a distance away and can be difficult to reach on public transport.
- As with all major cities, Manchester does have a higher than average crime rate and insurance premiums can be high.
- It has a habit of raining!

Further information

Manchester
Ms L M Harding
Admissions Officer
Faculty of Medicine
Stopford Building
University of Manchester
Oxford Road
Manchester M13 9PT
Tel: 0161 275 2077 (general admissions)
      0161 275 5994 (medical school)
Fax: 0161 275 5584
Email: ug.admissions@man.ac.uk
Web: http://www.man.ac.uk

Keele
Admissions and Recruitment Office
School of Medicine
Keele University
Staffordshire ST5 5BG
Tel: 01782 583 632/642
Fax: 01782 583 634
Email: medicine@keele.ac.uk
Web: http://www.keele.ac.uk

Preston
Dr Simon Wallis
Director of Medical Education and Hospital Dean
Tel: 01257 245 600
Email: simon.wallis@LTHTR.nhs.uk

Additional application information

Average A-level requirements	• AAB including chemistry
Average Scottish Higher requirements	• AAAAB
Graduate entry requirements	• 2:1 degree
Make-up of interview panel	• A chairperson and three others to include healthcare professionals and bioscientists
Months in which interviews are held	• November–April
Proportion of overseas students	• 6% at Manchester (until 2007 Keele can only consider applications from home and EU students)
Proportion of mature students	• 10%
Proportion of graduate students	• 10%
Faculty's view of students taking a gap year	• Acceptable if used constructively
Proportion of students taking intercalated degrees	• 5%
Possibility of direct entrance to clinical phase	• No
Fees for overseas students	• Check directly with medical school
Fees for graduates	• £1125
Ability to transfer to other medical schools	• Students are welcome to intercalate at other universities where the same learning opportunity
Assistance for elective funding	• Prizes and bursaries available are updated annually on the Manchester Medical School website
Assistance for travel to attachments	• GP placements are usually within 10 miles of your base hospital and information about public transport to each place is sent out with your placement pack
Access and hardship funds	• As for electives
Weekly rent	• £30–£50
Pint of lager	• £2 upward
Cinema	• £3–£5
Nightclub	• £5 upward

Newcastle and Durham (Queens Campus, Stockton)

	Newcastle		Durham
Key facts	Undergraduate	Graduate	Undergraduate
Course length	5 years	4 years	2 years at Durham then 3 years at Newcastle
Total number of medical undergraduates	1100	25	190
Applicants in 2003	2500	750	591
Interviews given in 2003	820	80	321
Places available in 2003	315	25	95
Places available in 2004	315	25	95
Open days 2004	30 June	30 June	April
Entrance requirements	AAB	2:1 Hons	AAB or 2:1
Mandatory subjects	Chemistry or biology at A- or AS-level	Degree in any discipline	All Phase I
Male:female ratio	60:40	50:50	45:65
Is an exam included in the selection process? If yes, what form does this exam take?	No	No	No
Qualification gained	MBBS		

Newcastle is a friendly city and the university is very centrally situated. The medical school is 5 minutes away from the main campus and is very near to the halls of residence. As in the rest of the university, there is a diversity of students, both national and international, from many different backgrounds. The staff are generally approachable and supportive, and well liked by students. Building work continues and the medical school is proud to have a brand new, state-of-the-art 400-seat lecture theatre and a "starship enterprise" entrance foyer.

At Newcastle, early patient contact comes from hospital and GP visits in the first two years, and the course attempts to break down the traditional preclinical/clinical divide. There are opportunities for extended contact with patients by way of the "family" and "chronic illness patient" studies (see below). The medical school is well established and highly regarded. Its graduates find that they are well placed to get the jobs they want, and, although many students choose to spread their wings after qualifying, many also choose to stay in the North East or to come back there later in their careers. The social life, centred on both the university and the city itself, is excellent, with something to appeal to everyone. Newcastle, the northernmost English university city, gives a warm welcome to its students.

In addition to the traditional 5-year medical degree at Newcastle, there is now the opportunity for graduates to apply for the accelerated 4-year course at Newcastle. This is a demanding course but has the obvious advantage of being a fast track to qualification.

The new medical school at Durham University is based at Queens Campus Stockton (some 20 miles from Durham, and 40 from Newcastle) in brand new facilities set along the regenerated Tees riverside. As the result of a partnership between Durham and Newcastle Universities, Stockton students spend the first 2 years of their Newcastle medical degree being taught at this campus as members of Durham University before being transferred and integrated with the much larger numbers of Newcastle students in years 3–5. The course in Stockton has been developed alongside that in Newcastle and aims to produce a cohort of students with the same levels of skills and knowledge as those produced via the more traditional route in Newcastle. Although the two courses work to similar terminal objectives, there are some key differences on the Durham course, which we have highlighted in the profile. Stockton is a small and friendly place and the town centre is only 10 minutes' walk from Queens campus. Although it might not boast all the attractions of a traditional university city, it has all the facilities you would expect of a big town, and, as Queens campus has become more established, it has become student-friendly with new café-bars and clubs, and an international summer arts festival. For nights out partying, then Middlesbrough is on the doorstep.

Durham University at Queens Campus has developed strong links with schools and colleges of education in the local area through a programme of open days and visits. It promotes a "widening access" policy, the benefits of which can be seen in its non-traditional student intake. Its medical students have qualifications ranging from the usual three science A-levels to first and second degrees in arts as well as sciences, and professional qualifications from worlds as diverse as law and nursing. Mature students are well represented and their presence has contributed to a genuinely interactive style of teaching with staff that is less didactic and more open to discussion than in many medical schools.

Students who start at either Newcastle or Durham quickly develop affection for their communities, whether it is the vibrant Newcastle or the rapidly developing campus at Stockton. At both centres, the large student presence makes for an excellent social life.

Education 🏴

The courses at Newcastle and Stockton are divided into two major phases based on the traditional preclinical/clinical model.

In Phase I (years 1 and 2) the course is case-led and systems-based, with an emphasis on a clinical approach from the start. There are several opportunities for early patient contact in the form of project work (a family study of a pregnant mother and her baby and a study of a patient with a chronic illness), and hospital and GP visits. Clinical skills are introduced, but just to give a flavour of relevance to the systems being studied. However, communication skills are given a high priority from the very beginning. The systems that the course covers include cardiovascular, respiratory, renal, gastrointestinal, endocrine, and the metabolism in year 1. In year 2 clinical sciences and investigative medicine are taught, with immunology, haematology, and neuromuscular skeletal systems. In both years, personal and professional development and medicine in the community are taught alongside. There are differences between the Newcastle and Stockton Phase 1. At Stockton, students do a 60-hour community placement in a local voluntary sector organisation and are assessed on this in year 2. In addition, the Stockton students are required to maintain a personal and professional development portfolio over their 2 years at Stockton and they undergo an interview on this before moving on to Phase 2. These aspects of the course reflect a greater emphasis on the social and cultural aspects of medicine at Stockton. A more traditional curriculum in Newcastle in the first 2 years presents the students with more emphasis on science-based subjects such as medical genetics in year 1, and a larger medical school means the Newcastle students have more consistent training in clinical skills in their first 2 years.

The accelerated course, which is available only in Newcastle, not Stockton, aims to combine the essential elements of years 1 and 2 into one intensive year. It achieves this by teaching core material over a 45-week year (rather than 2 years of 31 weeks) during which time a problem-based learning method is largely used. Lots of tutor support is available with students being taught in groups of 8–10. This accelerated Phase I began to run for the first time in 2002, and feedback from the students has been very positive.

With the creation of the accelerated Phase I, and the Stockton Phase I, which started only in 2001, the outcomes for the different entry routes have yet to be seen. However, it can be said that medicine in Newcastle is now being taken by a much more diverse population of students than ever before. In September 2003, the Newcastle Phase II (years 3, 4, and 5) contained for the first time Stockton students and accelerated course students, all brought together as one cohort.

Teaching

Phase 1 teaching is lecture-based (40–50% of the time) for the Newcastle and Stockton students, except for the accelerated course students, who follow a pattern of structured tutorials and anatomy classes with prosected specimens followed by self-directed study. All students on Phase 1 have small-group seminar work, practical sessions, clinical skills sessions, and self-directed study.

Both universities protect Wednesday afternoon from teaching to allow time for sport, art, and leisure (or just plain sleeping) across the universities.

In Phase II the students are allocated for their entire year 3 to a base unit, which consists of a cluster of hospitals located within the sizeable northern region as follows:

- **Teeside** (Middlesbrough, Stockton, Bishop Auckland, Darlington, Hartlepool)
- **Wear** (Sunderland, Durham, South Tyneside)
- **Tyne** (Newcastle hospitals and the Queen Elizabeth Hospital in Gateshead)
- **Northumbria** (North Tyneside, Ashington, Hexham, and Carlisle).

There is a degree of choice over which base unit students are allocated to, and most students end up with their first or second choice. Extenuating circumstances may guarantee a particular base unit, but for the majority of students decisions have to be made about whether to try to hold out for one of the closer hospitals or whether to opt for a more distant one. There are advantages to both. Almost all students opt to commute rather than stay in hospital accommodation where possible.

Phase II sees the emphasis shift significantly to clinical experience. There is an introductory "Foundations of Clinical Practice" course, lasting 16 weeks, which introduces students systematically and thoroughly to clinical history taking and examination, and is one of the best received parts of the course by students. After this, students embark on a series of essential junior rotations, which takes them through to the end of year 3. Students spend time in reproductive and child health, chronic illness and rehabilitation, mental health, public health, and infectious diseases. Throughout the year students spend one morning a week with a GP practice, which many students say is the highlight of the week as they have the opportunity to work in small groups of three and get a very individual and personalised experience.

Year 4 starts with another 16-week block, this time in "Clinical skills and investigative medicine", based back at Newcastle (the first direct experience of Newcastle University for some of the Stockton students).This is then followed by three 7-week student-selected modules (SSMs), and at the end of the year 4 by the 9-week elective period (to which 2 weeks' holiday can be added to extend your trip away).

The final year 5 consists of essential senior rotations in the major clinical specialties; acute and chronic hospital care, primary care, critical care, and mental health. Placements can be throughout the north from the west coast of Cumbria to Northumberland and down as far as Teeside. Final-year students spend five days a week in hospital and are expected to become part of the team to which they are attached, including being around during some evenings. The emphasis is on taking responsibility for your own self-directed learning, and therefore time is often left deliberately unstructured.

In terms of actual teaching, different students prefer different teaching styles, and there is something for everyone at Newcastle/Durham. For the first 2 years a student should consider carefully the various Phase I options, all of which have quite a different emphasis. A mature or local student might prefer the community spirit of Stockton. Someone coming straight from school and wanting to be at the heart of the action might think Newcastle is more their scene. Either way it is important to make the choice carefully because it may determine a student's feelings about where they want to be in year 3. After that students start to be directed by what they want to choose to study themselves in year 4, and then they head into their final preparation for working as a doctor in year 5.

Assessment

Phase I exams consist of a multiple-choice paper (MCQs), a data interpretation/problem solving paper, and a clinical-based objective structured clinical exam (OSCE). In Phase I exams are mid-year, and at the end of the year; and about 6 weeks into year 1 there is a short exam, which gives students a chance to see how they are progressing. There are also several in-course assessments which include essays, literature reviews, project work, presentations, and posters, as well as the SSMs.

Phase II exams consist of data interpretation/problem-solving papers, MCQs, and OSCEs. In-course assessment is by way of in-course marks for the junior rotations and SSMs in year 4. Final exams at the end of year 5 consist of data interpretation/problem-solving, an OSCE, and a "long case".

In all exams, there are vivas for borderline or distinction students.

Intercalated degrees

Students may wish to intercalate after either years 2 or 4. This means they study for a further year for the additional degree of BSc in various science subjects (Newcastle), or BSc Health and Human Sciences (Durham). They then slot back into their medical degree the following year, joining the year behind them. In addition, students can intercalate for a research masters or an MPhil at the end of year 4. Research projects available in intercalated years are wide ranging, from clinical to laboratory-based work, and topics in the social sciences. Until recently, at Newcastle, intercalation led to a BMedSci. It is not yet known how the change to BSc will affect the number of students wanting to intercalate. Traditionally about 10% took this route.

Special study modules and electives

Student-selected modules or special study modules, SSMs for short, in year 4 can be followed virtually anywhere across the northern region. It is also possible for students with a burning interest in a particular subject to set up an SSM themselves. As long as it is with the university's approval, it can be within the region or beyond. For those who don't want to go to the trouble of this, there are over 300 modules on offer by the university, some hospital-based, some community, and some in investigative medicine.

Electives are entirely up to the individual to plan and arrange. The university has a database of information from previous student electives, but the idea is to think creatively, and be adventurous if you wish.

Erasmus

There is no formal Erasmus programme in the medical school, but options exist to do languages as SSMs and to use these on electives, for example.

Facilities

Library   The Newcastle Medical Library is situated within the medical school and is open in the evenings during the week, but at more limited hours at weekends. It is well stocked with books and videos, but does get busy at exam time. Students may also use the university library, which is close to the medical school (5 minutes' walk). Durham students have full use of the Newcastle library facilities.

There are more limited library facilities at Stockton, where emphasis is put on using web-based resources such as MedLine in addition to textbook resources.

Computers   These tend to be very good, and much information is passed on to students via email. Computer courses are held as part of the course, specifically in word-processing and the use of email/internet to search databases.

There are well over 100 PCs at Newcastle Medical School, 10 of which are library-based. If all of these are busy, there are numerous quieter clusters throughout the university, which medical students can access.

Stockton has 200 computers on campus, with a significant number being library-based. All facilities at the university in Durham itself are available to Stockton students, as well as the Newcastle University facilities.

Clinical skills   The well-equipped clinical skills laboratories at Newcastle and Stockton are available for private revision as well as for timetabled teaching sessions.

Welfare

Student support

All students are assigned a personal tutor for pastoral support, and faculty staff are friendly and approachable. Both universities and Students' Unions have welfare officers and counselling services, including Nightline. All fresher medics join a peer family (often with five generations!) to help get them orientated. Those at UDSC have peer families in Newcastle as well, to encourage integration of the courses.

Mature students have an increasing presence at the medical school. Newcastle University has a mature students officer for advice on issues like finance and childcare and at Stockton free kids' club places are available during half-term holidays.

Accommodation

Newcastle freshers' accommodation is guaranteed in halls or self-catering flats, although not all are centrally located. The housing office offers help and advice to students renting in the private sector, as most do from year 2. Popular student areas for renting are Jesmond, Heaton, and Fenham. Renting is easy and cheap in Newcastle compared to many other universities.

At Stockton, most first-year students choose to live in halls which are all within 5 minutes of the medical department, and which offer an outstanding standard of accommodation because of the newness of the buildings. Most rooms have internet access, and prices are reasonable. In year 2 students tend to live out. Stockton has a lot of low-priced but reasonable quality accommodation, close to the university.

Placements

The Newcastle campus is situated very close to the city centre and includes the Royal Victoria Infirmary (adjoining the medical school). The facilities within the medical school are good – even including a gym. In the first 2 years, students will visit hospitals close to the medical school, but all the lecture-based teaching takes place at the medical school. This gives cohesiveness to the first 2 years which students appreciate.

At Stockton the smaller numbers lead to good opportunities for integration with both other Stockton students and those from the rest of Durham University. In the first 2 years, the majority of the teaching is based at the medical school, but some courses are taught in hospital teaching centres in the Tees and Durham area hospitals. This is generally enjoyed by the students who get to experience teaching from a vast number of clinicians in a range of different hospital and primary care settings from the very beginning. Travel expenses for the students are not refunded by either university for Stockton students in Phase I.

During Phase II, attachments may be much further afield such as at the base units in year 3. There is usually accommodation available in hospitals if students wish. Reimbursement of travel expenses is limited.

Students often find that the inconvenience of commuting to distant attachments is often outweighed by the fact that the smaller district general hospitals further afield usually have fewer students than the central teaching hospitals. The welcome given to students and the commitment to quality of teaching is generally excellent.

Sports and social 🏆

City life

Newcastle is a very lively city within easy reach of the hills of Northumberland and the unspoilt northeast coast of England. In recent years, Newcastle was voted eighth best "party" town in the world, with no shortage of bars and pubs, and an ever-increasing club scene. The medical school has good access to the city centre shops, theatre, cinema, museums, art galleries, and music venues. More shops are to be found at the Metrocentre, just across the River Tyne in Gateshead. The locals are generally very friendly and eager for everyone to have a good time. Stockton is nestled between the bustle of Middlesbrough and historic Durham, with easy access to both, and to other

Location of clinical placement/name of hospital	Distance away from Newcastle medical school	Difficulty getting there on public transport*	Accommodation available
Newcastle	2–4	+	No
Durham	18	++	No
Ashington	18	+++	No
Carlisle	50	+++	Yes
Middlesbrough	45	+++	Yes

*Ease of accessibility. +, set your alarm clock early; ++, long journey; +++, car is a must

cities in the north east. In Middlesbrough, pubs and clubs abound, and you can quickly get out to beautiful coast and moors of North Yorkshire. It is just as easy to visit the world heritage site of Durham Cathedral and lunch in one of the cosy cafés tucked away in Durham's narrow streets. In Stockton itself, there is a shopping complex with a multiplex cinema and bowling alley just minutes from the campus, and many student bars and nightclubs throughout the town.

University life

MedSoc is a great melting pot of all the years in the medical school and provides an opportunity to meet up with friends every week. MedSoc events take place in Newcastle every Friday evening, and usually consist of a guest speaker or show followed by a free bar. Previous events include karaoke nights and even a blind date evening. The annual MedSoc–DentSoc challenge is a regular favourite. Other highlights include the "Metro line" pub-crawl and exotic trips away to far-flung foreign cities like Edinburgh. Stockton's MedSoc has been up and running for 3 years now and has quite a repertoire of events held throughout the year.

The third-years annually stage a Medics' Revue in May, and there are numerous medics' balls and dinners throughout the year. The medics' summer ball is organised by the Newcastle Medical and Dental Student Council which is a student committee primarily concerned with support and welfare for medics and dentists. It is this organisation, which runs the peer-parenting scheme and organises events to support a wide range of charitable organisations.

Other organisations such as MedSin provide a campaigning link to international medical student organisations like The International Federation of Medical Students Associations (IFMSA); dedicated students forge links with the community, working with local schools providing sex education for example, and with disadvantaged groups such as asylum seekers. Regular student BMA meetings are held for those students politically minded.

A huge range of other clubs and societies are available through the Students Unions of both universities.

Sports life

At Newcastle, medics' rugby, netball, and hockey teams compete in leagues, and there are also football, volleyball, cricket, squash, and other sports clubs for medics, and innumerable other university-run clubs. The medical school in Newcastle has its own gym (£7 per year), and the university sports facilities are good and close by (around £50 per year).

At Stockton there is a great deal of interest in sport at all levels with rowing and canoeing being very popular, making use of the nearby Tees Barrage canoeing facilities. Sport in Durham is taken seriously at college and university levels.

For the enthusiastic spectator there are Newcastle, Middlesbrough, and Sunderland Football Clubs locally as well as rugby, basketball, athletics, cross-country, and more.

Fascinating fact: Newcastle Medical School might have expanded with the creation of its link with Durham, but in fact, the medical school started in Durham. In a moment of insanity about 50 years ago Durham actually gave it away to Newcastle, and regretted it ever since.

Great things about Newcastle

- The locals are friendly – adding to this vibrant, rapidly developing city where the atmosphere is never impersonal.
- Cost of living is relatively low.
- If you need a break from city life, it is easy to escape to the country or the coast.
- New pubs, clubs, and restaurants spring up all the time, with the Quayside and Jesmond being student favourites.
- Free beer at MedSoc (for life!).

Bad things about Newcastle

- There is some trepidation about how the increase in student numbers in recent years might affect course organisation and the student body.
- Travelling around the region can be time consuming without a car and costly with one.
- Timetable planning is sometimes communicated to students late.
- The tutor system doesn't work for everyone and so the amount of pastoral support students receive is variable.
- Some consultants mutter bitter words to the effect of "Of course, the students at Newcastle don't know any anatomy these days." You'll get sick of hearing it!

Great things about Durham (Queens campus, Stockton)

- Brand new state-of-the-art facilities, with very committed staff.
- Small (190 medical students in the department in total).

- Most of the teaching is delivered by a wide range of clinicians who come from many different hospitals and primary care centres in the region.
- Access to both Durham and Newcastle University facilities, for example, libraries.
- Patient-centred course with high emphasis on communication skills.

Bad things about Durham (Queens campus, Stockton)

- The library is noisy and lacks the comprehensive stock of a more established medical school library.
- The number of staff permanently in the medical school is very small.
- Stockton is a small town.
- The transition for Stockton students to Newcastle's curriculum in Phase II is not yet fully tried and tested.
- The aims of the partnership between Durham and Newcastle are a fudge. The big question is, "When will Durham go it alone?".

Further information

The Medical School
University of Newcastle
Framlington Place
Newcastle Upon Tyne NE2 4HH
Tel: 0191 222 7005
Fax: 0191 222 621
Email: admission-enquiries@ncl.ac.uk
Web: http://www.ncl.ac.uk
http://medical.faculty.ncl.ac.uk/undergrad/medicine

University of Durham
Phase 1 Medicine
School for Health
Queens Campus Stockton University
Boulevard
Stockton-on-Tees TS17 6BH
Tel: 0191 334 2000 (main switchboard)
Web: http://www.dur.ac.uk/phase1.medicine/

Additional application information

	Newcastle	Durham
Average A-level requirements	AAB, must include chemistry and/or biology. The school also requires at least AAAAB at GCSE, including maths, science, and English language	
Average Scottish Higher requirements	Contact college admissions directly for further information	
Graduate entry requirements	2:1 in any discipline	
Make-up of interview panel	Two members from a pool of academic and clinical staff and lay members	
Months in which interviews are held	November–March	
Proportion of overseas students	6%	0%
Proportion of mature students	10%	30%
Faculty's view of students taking a gap year	Positive	Positive
Proportion of students taking intercalated degrees	9%	Not yet known
Possibility of direct entrance to clinical phase	No	N/A
Fees for overseas students	c £10 000–£18 000	N/A
Fees for graduates	£1125	£1125
Ability to transfer to other medical schools	Not unheard of, but rare. Depends on personal circumstance, among other things	
Assistance for elective funding	Students can apply for a bursary if in financial difficulty	
Assistance for travel to attachments	Limited help, none from Durham. Also LEA/ELB/SAAS	
Access and hardship funds	Available, but don't bank on them	
Weekly rent	£40–60	
Pint of lager	£2.00 at Tiger Tiger on a Saturday night, and £1.50 in the Union	
Cinema	£3.95	
Nightclub	£1.00–£3.00 in the week. More at weekends	

Nottingham and Derby

Nottingham

	Nottingham ↓	Derby ↓
Key facts	Undergraduate	Graduate
Course length	5 years	4 years
Total number of medical undergraduates	c 1200	
Applicants in 2003	2400	1300
Interviews given in 2003	900	200
Places available in 2003	245	91
Places available in 2004	245	91
Open days 2004	20 and 21 June	17 April
Entrance requirements	AAB	2:2 Hons or better in any discipline
Mandatory subjects	Biology and chemistry	None
Male:female ratio	40:60	55:45
Is an exam included in the selection process? If yes, what form does this exam take?	No	Yes, GAMSAT
Qualification gained	BMedSci and BMBS	

Nottingham is a campus university with a community atmosphere in a vibrant city. Medics and non-medics mix in year 1 in superb halls of residence on a beautiful campus built around a lake. There is plentiful off-campus accommodation, mostly located in the Lenton area between the campus and the city. This area is very student-orientated, so that many friends will live within walking distance of each other throughout the course. The cost of living compares favourably with other university towns, and the city is very multicultural. The medical school is a part of the massive Queen's Medical Centre (QMC) hospital at the city end of the university campus. The course is systems-based, with emphasis on the early introduction of clinical skills. Outside placements are accessible and the quality of teaching is high. All students do a BMedSci degree within the 5-year course, and there are growing opportunities to study abroad. Clinical attachments are assessed individually and within themselves. The elective follows finals and this works very well, allowing less worry and more knowledge. Most graduates choose to find PRHO jobs through the matching scheme and stay in the Nottingham area.

Education

Nottingham offers a blend between traditional and modern-style courses. Throughout the 5 years the subjects are split into four themes: cell, body, community, and communication/social – learn this for the interview!

The first 2 years are integrated clinically, with systems-based teaching arranged in four semesters. One morning every fortnight is spent seeing patients, either in general practice or in hospital, and clinical skills are taught and examined in both years.

Year 3 is split into two halves: the first involves a research project leading to a BMedSci degree for everybody; the second marks the beginning of full-time clinical study, with general medical and surgical attachments after a brief introductory course.

The final 2 years are spent on clinical attachments in a variety of specialties such as paediatrics, obstetrics and gynaecology and psychiatry, before returning to general medicine and surgery. Throughout the course, there is a large but appropriate emphasis on personal and professional development; this includes communication skills, ethics, and career advice.

Teaching

Lectures form the basis of most first- and second-year modules, and the main lecture theatres were renovated earlier this year, with new comfy seats. Lectures are supplemented with a limited number of tutorials (about 10 students) and seminars (about 25 students). Anatomy is taught by group dissection (10 students) and clinical problem-solving in the newly renovated dissection laboratories. Practical classes are taught in large telelinked laboratories.

Assessment

The course is examined by continual assessment instead of a single final exam after the 5 years. Depending on your outlook, this either reduces or spreads the inevitable stress. In years 1 and 2 exams take place in January and June, often using MCQs, ie negatively marked true and false questions (these can be more challenging than they sound). The BMedSci is assessed mainly from a 10 000–15 000-word research-based project. In the clinical years, logbook assessment and practical exams follow each attachment, with MCQ exams twice a year. In year 5, the finals are clinically orientated, involving medicine, surgery, orthopaedics, and clinical laboratory sciences; the year was redesigned recently to allow several practice attempts at finals before the real exam.

Intercalated degrees

Despite this being a 5-year course, everyone does a research-based BMedSci (Hons) degree in year 3. The exam results of the first 2 years contribute 50% of the final degree mark. Students who leave the course after this have the benefit of a degree qualification. This is a comfort, but not many students leave mid-course. Many students use their projects to publish scientific papers or present them at conferences. These projects usually involve hard work but provide excellent analytical and self-directed learning skills for clinicals. The BMedSci projects are distributed in a lottery style fashion and so you have limited control over what you eventually research. However, most students enjoy the experience.

Special study modules and electives

The 8-week elective is at the end of all clinical attachments and the final exams in year 5. However, if you have failed any clinical examinations in years 4 and 5, you may have to resit them in this period. Most people choose a mixture of work and play, although a short report is expected from everyone. Earlier in year 5 there are two 5-week long SSMs. The variety of choices are good and Nottingham currently offers 30 SSM places throughout Europe.

Erasmus

A limited number of students have had the opportunity to complete their BMedSci project overseas. This is dependent on which department you are placed in and whether such an opportunity is available that year. In the paediatrics and the obstetrics and gynaecology attachment, there is an opportunity to complete this module abroad in a Scandinavian country. Again, places are limited and so competition is fierce.

Facilities

Library   The medical library is on the ground floor of the medical school; it is large and the staff are friendly. It is well stocked with core texts and journals, but can become busy around exam times. It opens until 11.15 pm weekdays, and during the day at weekends for most of the year.

Computers   IT facilities are good, with over 200 terminals in the medical school. There is unlimited and free access to email, the internet, teaching CD ROMs, and computer-assisted learning packages for teaching and revision. The recently redesigned Networked Learning Environment allows internet access to lecture handouts, slides, and learning aids from outside the medical school. The main computer room is open 24 hours a day. Facilities at outlying hospitals are improving.

Clinical skills   There are a series of newly built rooms dedicated to teaching clinical skills, such as examining patients. The laboratory is staffed and resources have rapidly grown to an excellent level. It is used on a casual basis and has many self-teaching aids – suturing practice kits, models of eyes, ears, arms (for blood pressure), videos, etc.

Welfare

Student support

As a whole the university has a friendly feel and student welfare is taken very seriously. In the medical school every student is allocated a tutor who can address academic or personal problems. Unfortunately, the amount of "actual" support given varies from tutor to tutor. The students organise a mentoring system in which first-years are allocated individual second-year "parents". Whether or not you meet regularly with your "parent" depends on how well you get on; however, a high rate of adoption and incest leaves most people happy! The university and Students' Union have welfare, legal, financial, and counselling services, along with an active Niteline (night-time counselling service) run by students.

Accommodation

Almost all first-years are housed in good-quality university accommodation; these are mostly catered halls, though some students opt for self-catering flats. There are 12 medium-sized halls on the main campus, each with its own bar. A further three large halls are found on the recently built Jubilee campus, about 15 minutes' walk from the main campus or QMC. In subsequent years you can apply to stay in halls, though most students move into private rented houses: 80% choose to live in Lenton, which is a relatively safe student area, 20 minutes' walk from the campus and town. House hunting begins very early after Christmas; most students organise it themselves without university vetting. The Union organises house-hunting for first-years wanting to live out before their first term.

Placements

The teaching hospitals are all located within one rush-hour drive of Nottingham. The smaller hospitals are generally friendlier (as they have more time to talk to you), but sometimes more work is expected from you. Accommodation is provided free of charge in Mansfield and Lincoln depending on which placement you are doing. Otherwise, you are expected to travel daily.

Clinical visits in years 1 and 2 often require some travelling, but transport or suggested routes are provided. Students usually organise to share car lifts as some hospitals can be very difficult to travel to on public transport.

Sports and social

City life

The city centre is attractive, compact, and has good shopping facilities. Nottingham is renowned for its inexpensive and diverse bars, clubs, pubs, and restaurants. The theatres are good, but there are

Location of clinical placement/name of hospital	Distance away from medical school (miles)	Difficulty getting there on public transport*	Accommodation available
Queens Medical Centre	0	+	No
Nottingham City Hospital	5	+	No
Derby General Hospital	25	++	No
Mansfield Hospital	30	++	Yes
Lincoln Hospital	45	+++	Yes

*Ease of accessibility: +, set your alarm clock early; ++; long journey; +++, car is a must

few live music venues. The city centre is within walking distance of most off-campus accommodation, and a 10-minute bus ride (£1) from campus. Because of its central location, travel to most other cities is quick and easy. The Peak District and surrounding countryside provide a welcome escape where students can enjoy themselves, far away from anatomy revision.

University life

Student life is rich and varied, and there is plenty of time to enjoy it while doing a medical degree. The student medical society (MedSoc) provides a good range of social events (eg cocktail parties), balls, and guest lectures. MedSin is also very active in Nottingham, so it is easy to get involved in projects such as Sexpression, WaterAid, Heartstart, and Marrow. Nottingham has one of the largest student rags in the country, called *Karni*. This raises about £230 000 for charity from activities in the first term. On-campus entertainment revolves around hall life, and includes bars and themed parties. In later years the pub and club scenes of Lenton and the city dominate. There are also hundreds of university clubs and societies facilitating much interaction within the student body from Unifilms to MutantSoc!

The main distinguishing feature of Nottingham medics' social life is the extent to which medical students are mixed with the whole university population. After year 1, many medics live with their non-medic friends from halls. Lenton, the main student area, is well equipped with cheapish pubs, launderettes, late-opening shops, take-aways, video rental shops, and buses. Although the campus accommodation is excellent, the university could take more responsibility for off-campus housing.

Sports life

Nottingham has good quality, accessible sporting facilities including a swimming pool on campus. Medics' teams play against the hall teams; they are particularly strong in hockey, rugby, tennis, and football. Most sports and standards of ability are represented somewhere in the university. The clubs provide a focus for excellent social lives.

Fascinating fact: Emeritus Professor Sir Peter Mansfield designed the first MRI scanner at Nottingham. He has just received the Nobel Prize for his pioneering work.

Derby

The Graduate Entry Medicine (GEM) course at Derby is situated in a new, purpose-designed, medical school on the grounds of the Derby City General Hospital (DCGH). Entrants can be graduates of any discipline and students study for 18 months in Derby and then proceed onto the same 30 months of clinical training that students at Nottingham receive. Successful students graduate with BMBS degrees from The University of Nottingham. The brand new building provides a comfortable learning environment and, being based on a hospital site, gives a sense of vocation.

- Length of course: 4 years
- Applicants for 2003 entry: 1240
- Annual intake: 90 students
- Entry requirements: a 2:2 degree (any discipline); successful GAMSAT result; 45 minutes interview.

Education

The mainstay of education, during the preclinical months, is problem-based learning (PBL). Each week the problem changes and the groups discuss a new medical topic. These sessions are good fun but require a great deal of self-directed learning if they are to be effective. Lectures, specific to the current problem, accompany the PBL topic of the week. PBL topics are divided into successive blocks: foundation, musculoskeletal, respiratory, cardiovascular, endocrine and nutrition, renal, alimentary, cancer, and neurosciences. Anatomy, related to the current PBL topic, is taught by lectures and prosection. Personal and Professional Development (PPD) is composed of clinical skills workshops, lectures and GP placements. Clinical skills workshops teach basic procedures, such as auscultation and taking blood pressure, as well as communication. There are nine GP placements during the preclinical months. The clinical months are as described for Nottingham.

Teaching

This is by highly experienced staff: many of whom are practising clinicians and there is a strong clinical emphasis to the teaching. Some academics travel from Nottingham to lecture.

Assessment

After the first 18 months of the course, PBL is assessed with a set of final written exams. Students also do an objective structured clinical examination (OSCE) at this time. PPD is assessed with a portfolio review at the end of year 1. At the end of each PBL block a formative exam is set; the results of this are for personal use only and do not contribute to the final degree mark. The clinical years, the final 30 months of the course, are assessed as described for students at the University of Nottingham.

Intercalated degrees

These are not available as all students are already graduates.

Facilities

Access to the building is available 24 hours a day, 7 days a week. Only the library, lecture theatre, seminar room, clinical skills centre and anatomy suite have set hours of access. Walk-in access is available to anatomical learning aids throughout the day. Each group of seven or eight students has exclusive access, via a key code, to their own PBL room. Each room is equipped with two computers, tables, white boards, lockers and a set of core textbooks. Students also have their own common room with pool table and veranda.

Library The new library is very well stocked with the latest editions of many texts. All of the core texts are multiple-stocked in both the short and weeklong loan sections. There are few paper journals held but online access is available for most. Photocopying facilities and 10 computers, linked to a printer, are available. The library is open until 9.45 pm on weeknights and is open at the weekends. Derby campus students have full access to the Greenfield Medical Library, at the QMC in Nottingham, and may use the library of the Derby City General Hospital. There is a public library in the city centre.

Computers There are 54 computers in the main computer room and six computers in the smaller one. There is also a laser printer and quiet work desks. All computers in the building are linked to the University of Nottingham network with fast broadband internet access. Most lecture PowerPoint presentations are available from the GEM website, along with a vast amount of learning resources. The PBL scenarios, and all associated learning materials, can also be found here. Email is widely used for communication within the school, along with the bulletin board on the GEM website. Access is available to the computers at all times.

Clinical skills Booking is available for extra practice with equipment in the clinical skills centre.

Welfare

Student support

The staff at the school are friendly and on first name terms with students. Each student is assigned a personal mentor: a member of staff available to help with both personal and academic issues. Students meet with mentors at the end of each PBL block to formally review progress; this also gives the opportunity to raise concerns of any kind. Meetings are relaxed and staff are very approachable. All of the university and Students' Union services described for Nottingham are also available to Derby students.

Accommodation

Accommodation at Lonsdale Hall is available through the university. Lonsdale Hall is a large site of self-catered flats with seven to eight students sharing. Many students choose instead to share a house. There is a good availability of housing and private flats in the area.

Placements

These are the same as described for the Nottingham students.

Sports and social 🏆

City life

Derby has well-connected train and bus stations. A return bus ticket to Nottingham is either £2 or £6.50 depending on whether you want a 60- or 30-minute journey, respectively. All major high-street names can be found and there are almost as many banks as shops! There are many bars, some late licensed, and a few clubs, but generally, it is very lively. The medical school is about a 25-minutes' walk away from Lonsdale hall. A retail park, with a Sainsbury's, is a 15-minutes' walk from Lonsdale, and Tesco is within driving distance. Buses into the town centre from near the medical school or Lonsdale Hall are frequent and cost £1.60 return maximum; it is a 25-minutes' walk from Lonsdale. Parking near the medical school costs £52 for a permit that lasts a year. The surrounding area of Derbyshire is very beautiful and many people take up walking there.

University life

The university pays for affiliate membership of all students with the University of Derby Students' Union. This gives access to their societies and events. Students are automatically members of the University of Nottingham Students' Union but travelling can become tedious. A MedSoc, for social events, is currently being set up, along with an anatomy society.

Sports life

A variety of different medical student sports teams are currently being set up. However, students can use sporting facilities located near the university accommodation as well.

Great things about Nottingham 👍

- You get a bonus degree (BMedSci) without having to do an extra year; this is very useful later in your career.
- Good social life for students, with variety, value, and accessibility along with many active and friendly student societies.
- Beautiful campus, with good community spirit and healthy interhall rivalry.

- Integration of medics with non-medics in halls broadens social circles and reduces the cliquishness that medics are sometimes accused of!
- After year 1, all your hall friends remain within walking distance by moving to the student area (Lenton).

Bad things about Nottingham 👎

- Because of the poor Union bar and lack of a campus venue for top bands, there is little to attract medics back to campus after year 1.
- It is felt that the university attracts students of a similar background, leading to a lack of diversity within the student population.
- Experiences of the year 3 Honours project are very variable in terms of workload, expectations, and assessment.
- The preclinical course is too lecture-based.
- Nottingham tends to like using computer-matching schemes to allocate students to BMedSci projects, PRHO jobs, and other parts of the course. Students often feel as though they have little control over their future – it's almost like a lottery!

Great things about Derby 👍

- Attractive new purpose-designed building.
- Excellent teaching and facilities.
- Wide mix of students with different degrees and life experiences.
- Close community atmosphere.
- Much of the teaching is by clinicians.

Bad things about Derby 👎

- You can feel fairly isolated from the main university and Students' Union.
- Not many student societies are set up yet because the course is new.
- Everyone studies the same thing, so there is not much integration with other students.
- Small number of students means that you can get to know everyone perhaps too well!
- If you both work and live with medics, you can get "medicine overload syndrome".

Further information

Admissions Officer
Faculty Office
Queen's Medical Centre
University of Nottingham
Nottingham NG7 2RD
Tel: 0115 970 9379
Fax: 0115 970 9922
Email: medschool@nottingham.ac.uk
Web: http://www.nottingham.ac.uk

Additional application information	Nottingham	Derby (graduate course)
Average A-level requirements	• AAB at A-level, with grade As in biology and chemistry and a third subject (excluding general studies). At least 6 GCSEs passed at grade A to include the three sciences or the science double award, maths and English language passed at grade B or higher	
Average Scottish Higher requirements	• AB in chemistry and biology at Advanced Highers, plus two grade Bs in Highers	
Graduate entry requirements	• 2:2 Hons or better in any discipline	• 2:2 Hons or better in any discipline. Will accept a Masters or PhD in lieu of a first degree
Make-up of interview panel	• Two assessors comprising GPs, clinicians, academics	
Months in which interviews and held	• November–March	
Proportion of overseas students	• 10%	• 0% (Home, EU students only)
Proportion of mature students	• c 10%	
Proportion of graduate students	• c 10%	• 100%
Faculty's view of students taking a gap year	• Acceptable provided constructive	
Proportion of students taking intercalated degrees	• All students do a BMedSci year without doing an extra year	• 0%
Possibility of direct entrance to clinical phase	• No	• No
Fees for overseas students	• £9660 pa (years 1, 2) £17 730 pa (years 3, 4, and 5)	• £1125
Fees for graduates	• £1125	
Ability to transfer to other medical schools	• Yes, usually after completion of BMedSci degree in year 3. Individual circumstances are considered separately	
Assistance for elective funding	• Not directly, but students are invited to apply for elective prizes	
Assistance for travel to attachments	• No, students must apply to their LEA/ELB/SAAS and the medical school will validate your claim	
Access and hardship funds	• Yes, but some funds must be paid back later. All cases are dealt with anonymously	
Weekly rent	• Halls £40 (self-catering); £95 (fully catered); £45–£55 (private)	
Pint of lager	• Union bar £1.40; city centre pub £2.20	
Cinema	• Costs £4 with NUS student card	
Nightclub	• Free–£4, though posh clubs charge more at the weekends	

Oxford

Key facts	Undergraduate	Graduate
Course length	6 years	4 years
Total number of medical undergraduates	c 677	c 20
Applicants in 2003	941	280
Interviews given in 2003	823	100
Places available in 2003	150	30
Places available in 2004	150	30
Open days 2004	30 June, 1 July	Easter and Summer
Entrance requirements	AAA	2:1 or better GPA above 3.5
Mandatory subjects	Chemistry	Bioscience or chemistry degree
Male:female ratio	45:55	60:40
Is an exam included in the selection process? If yes, what form does this exam take?	Yes, two-hour test joint with Cambridge and UCL	Yes, two-hour written paper
Qualification gained	BM, BCh	BM, BCh

Oxford is a unique place. If you would like to live in either modern accommodation or 15th century halls and meet students of all backgrounds; have the double benefits of a small college and a large university; with a traditional yet innovative medical course, then Oxford is for you!

As with most medical schools the course has undergone some recent changes and the size of the school is gradually being increased by 50%. The recent addition of an accelerated course for bioscience graduates is another innovation.

Some may criticise the lack of clinical involvement during the first 3 years of the 6-year undergraduate course. However, the firm scientific basis of medicine is of vital importance and the acquisition of skills, such as the critical evaluation of papers and an understanding of research, is rightly given a very high priority. Three years before significant patient contact may seem like a long time to some, but the knowledge and skills gained during the preclinical course will be of use for the rest of your career, and having an "extra" science degree is no bad thing when applying for medical jobs.

The course demands the very highest level of academic ability and commitment. However, your college tutor, who selects you in the first place, has a vested interest in your success and, in most cases, works very hard on your behalf – no one is left to struggle. The short terms and long holidays also make the hard work survivable and enjoyable.

Education

Oxford Medical School was recently assessed by the QAA as a single 6-year course, but, for practical purposes, there remains a clear-cut division between the preclinical and clinical courses in Oxford. At present, in the preclinical school the first five terms are spent studying the basic medical sciences (anatomy, biochemistry, physiology, pathology, and neuroscience), and the final four terms working for an Honours degree. (The timetable for the first 2 years is currently under review, but the subjects will remain the same.) Application to the clinical school is competitive, with about 55–65% of the Oxford preclinical students staying on. The rest go mainly to London or Cambridge, and there is an influx of students from elsewhere – mainly Cambridge – with additions from London and the Scottish medical schools.

The clinical course lasts 3 years and aims to deliver the best teaching of both scientific principles and clinical practice. It is in a particularly good position to do so, because of the combination of its small size and the very high quality of its academic and clinical staff. Year 4 consists of medicine, surgery, and an 8-week laboratory medicine course (pathology), together with a residential general practice attachment, ethics, and communication skills. Special Study Modules (SSMs) are an exciting and innovative addition to year 4. These can be taken in subjects such as philosophy, theology, chronic illness, and creativity, where students are free to explore their particular interests. The year begins with an improved 5-week foundation course, a fortnight of which is dedicated to teaching from year 6 students. This allows a gentle transition from preclinical to clinical studies for the year 4 students while giving the final-year students a chance to teach.

Year 5 contains all the specialist rotations: paediatrics, obstetrics and gynaecology, A&E, orthopaedics, general practice, neurology, ENT, ophthalmology, and psychiatry. Year 6 focuses again on medicine and surgery (5 weeks each), with a 10-week elective period, 14 weeks of clinical special study modules, a 6-week PRHO shadowing at a district general hospital (DGH), and several revision weeks. Throughout the clinical course, there is a great deal of ward-based teaching, with both consultants and the junior doctors (all of whom are keen to practise being teaching hospital consultants!). The modular form of the specialist rotations means that there is no easy year 5, but the pressure at finals is much reduced. At present, as almost all the clinical students are in Oxford at any one time, there is a strong sense of group identity and a very full social life.

Teaching

In the preclinical years the basic medical sciences are taught by lectures and practicals, supported by most colleges giving tutorials with two to three students, two to three times a week. Teaching in the clinical years is ward- and clinic-based.

214

Assessment

Currently, the assessments are at the end of year 1 and before Easter in year 2, and consist of essay papers, short notes, and problem-solving questions. Practical skills are assessed continuously and practical books must be kept up to date.

Intercalated degrees

All students spend the last terms of the preclinical phase working for an Honours degree in physiology or psychology (unless they are already graduates). The degree course has a large amount of flexibility, and students are encouraged to follow courses that interest them.

Special study modules and electives

There is a 10-week elective in year 6 for which most students choose to go abroad. Some of the colleges can help financially. The 14 weeks of SSMs in the final year are more clinical in nature than the modules of the first clinical year. There are over 60 options, ranging from the traditional (such as cardiology, anaesthetics, and general practice), to the innovative (creativity in health care, medical publishing, medical anthropology, or even a language), and can be either purely clinical, research, or a mixture of both. If the extensive list does not cover the one subject that you desperately want to study, you are free, with the medical school's permission, to arrange your own. This can on occasion be undertaken outside Oxford and even abroad.

Erasmus

Whilst it is more challenging to arrange study abroad during the preclinical part of the course, there are plenty of travel opportunities during the clinical years. Year 5 placements in paediatrics and obstetrics and gynaecology can both be partly undertaken abroad. In addition, the 10-week elective scheme in the final year enables experience of medicine anywhere in the world. As well as these opportunities, it is possible to arrange an SSM in a foreign country (or partly abroad).

Facilities

Library   Oxford is very well catered for with respect to libraries. At preclinical level, the Radcliffe Science Library (RSL) and college libraries are the most useful and are well used. College facilities vary but, in general, are at a very high standard. The RSL has an incredible number of books and journals, but rather limited opening hours out of term time. The Cairns Library is located at the John Radcliffe Hospital, and is the library used during clinical years. It is very well stocked and opens 24 hours a day, 365 days a year.

Computers   The computing facilities are very good in colleges, departments, libraries and, at clinical level, in Osler House and the Cairns Library, where a large number of computers are reserved exclusively for medical students. Computer-assisted learning is soon to be introduced, and all lecture notes and resources for courses such as the laboratory medicine course, are available electronically.

Clinical skills   A laboratory currently exists and is used for medical and surgical skills teaching. From next year a new larger laboratory is due to be built and will be used to teach a more comprehensive list of skills required for use as a PRHO. An automated dummy (called Harvey!) has recently been purchased for skills teaching.

Welfare

Student support

Oxford students are considered to be friendly and very social. There is a niche for everyone. The university tutoring system works well in the preclinical years because of the collegiate system. In clinical years, when links with the college are not as strong, the system does not work so well but is supplemented by good support, be it academic or pastoral, from the medical school. Colleges provide significant financial assistance, ranging from subsidised accommodation, meals, and entertainment, to elective funding and hardship grants. Oxford University has welfare and counselling facilities, in addition to the provision by the medical school and colleges.

At preclinical and especially clinical levels, medical students tend to know each other very well. Depending on your viewpoint, this can either be an advantage or a disadvantage, but most seem to enjoy the camaraderie and banter, whether in the bar or in the dissection room! One of the great things about Oxford is the collegiate system: this broadens your horizons and makes it very easy to make friends with non-medics. At the clinical level, Osler House Club (the Students' Union) provides a very relaxed way of meeting people and making friends.

Accommodation

Preclinical students will find their life well integrated with that of students in other subjects and will live with them in college accommodation. Many of the college buildings are old and beautiful, but do bear in mind that sometimes the accommodation you will actually live in will either be 1950s or private lodgings. All the accommodation is of a reasonable to good or excellent standard, and fairly cheap.

Things are very different for clinical students, however. Very few live on college sites, as the majority of graduate accommodation is in nearby annexes. The exception is Green College, which was established for medical students and is still largely populated by them. Many prefer to live out during their clinical training, as it affords more independence than college can provide, and there is plenty of good-quality private accommodation in Oxford.

Placements

The early years are spent studying basic medical sciences in and around the centre of Oxford. This is amid the Oxford colleges, with their long traditions of study and learning. The clinical school is based at the John Radcliffe Hospital (JR), which is a large teaching hospital situated in Headington, 2 miles east of Oxford city centre and easily accessible by bus or bike. It is modern, large, and

Location of clinical placement/name of hospital	Distance away from medical school (miles)	Difficulty getting there on public transport*	Accommodation available
John Radcliffe	2	+	No
Banbury	27	+	Yes
Reading	27	++	Yes
Northampton	42	+++	Yes
Milton Keynes	39	+++	Yes

*Ease of accessibility: +, set your alarm clock early; ++, long journey; +++, car is a must

contains all of Oxford's acute medical and surgical services. The Churchill Hospital is increasingly becoming a specialist centre for certain services, such as transplants, oncology, and soon diabetes and endocrinology. The Radcliffe Infirmary contains services for neurology, ENT, ophthalmology, and plastic surgery. It is due to be closed down and relocated to the JR site within the next 5 years. The Nuffield Orthopaedic Hospital, and the Warneford and Littlemore psychiatric hospitals are smaller centres used for specific modules of the course. All the hospitals are easily reached by bike, bus, or car (although parking is almost impossible!).

Although other hospitals in Banbury, Reading, Swindon, Northampton, and Bath are used, the majority of a student's time will still be spent in Oxford. Many find this very useful, as it allows them to be involved in university and college life, whether sports, drama, music, or other activities. There are, however, many opportunities to travel (in addition to the elective) for those who want to: for example, several of the specialties (such as paediatrics, and deliveries in obstetrics) can be studied in other parts of the country or world.

Sports and social 🏆

City life

Oxford, the "city of dreaming spires", is a small city with easy access to the rest of the country, and London in particular (only 50 minutes by train and 90 minutes by coach). Many preclinical students survive the first 3 years without needing to travel more than 5 minutes on foot from the centre of the city, but at clinical school, you are forced to move a little further afield. The town centre has the usual core of shops, and you will find it sufficient for most needs. Having said that, it does not compare to most "real" cities for variety. Culturally there is a lot going on, particularly if you like theatre and music. It has to be said that the club scene in Oxford is not very exciting and wouldn't suit the more dedicated punter, but you can get to and from London on buses leaving every 12–15 minutes, 24 hours a day.

University life

There are numerous university- and college-based clubs and societies dedicated to ensuring that students get the most they can out of their time in Oxford. At preclinical level, these often form a prominent part of most people's social life, with the medical society (MedSoc) supplementing this. The societies range from the sublime to the ridiculous, and you will find that talents you never realised you had are catered for.

The clinical school social life tends to revolve around Osler House, a 1920s house in the grounds of the John Radcliffe Hospital run for and by clinical students. There is a bar, a television room, computing facilities, pool table, and a pleasant garden, with lunch served daily. The Osler Committee organises many events – social, sporting, and cultural; however, many clinical students also remain involved in other aspects of university life, be it at their college or elsewhere. The clinical school pantomime, *Tingewick*, deserves a special mention. This takes place every year and is a great chance for the students to get their own back at their consultants and anyone else who deserves parody.

Sports life

Oxford is famous for its rowing and rugby, but other sports are well represented too. In particular, the collegiate structure means that there are both facilities and opportunities for involvement in sport at any level of ability. All the colleges have sports pitches and boathouses, and many can provide squash and tennis courts as well. Intercollegiate competitions (Cuppers) form one focus for the competitive energy, and the very committed will find themselves competing at the highest levels – the Varsity competitions. Even if you lack speed, strength, skill, accuracy, or talent in general, you will still be able to find a team of your level and skill! In the collegiate events, the clinical school is represented by the Osler–Green teams, who regularly manage to field competitive sides.

Fascinating fact: One lucky person every year at the medical school will have the traditional honour of playing the rear end of a large pink elephant in the medical school pantomime!

Good things about Oxford

- The collegiate system – meeting students in a variety of subjects, which predisposes to broader interests and education.
- Tutorial system: having one-to-one or two-to-one tuition, with the academic support that this offers. Consequently, very few students fall behind in their work.
- The influx of up to 50 new students from other medical schools in year 4 creates a fantastic opportunity to make new friends when you begin your clinical training.
- Excellent scientific and clinical teaching, together with a stimulating environment in a university with a first-class, worldwide reputation.
- Oxford is a beautiful city in which to work and, together with its traditions, this makes Oxford a unique and rare experience.

Bad things about Oxford

- The public perception of Oxford is behind the times and relies too much on stereotypes. These are inaccurate and unhelpful – do not be discouraged from applying!
- Some students at Oxford are incredibly hard working, so the pressure can build up at times.
- The scientific nature of the course, particularly during the preclinical years, does not suit everyone.
- The nightlife in Oxford is limited, but London is nearby and easily reached.
- The PRHO matching scheme doesn't work well.

Further information

Oxford Colleges Admission Service (undergraduate admissions)
The University Offices
Wellington Square
Oxford OX1 2JD
Tel: 01865 270 207
Fax: 01865 270 208
Email: undergraduate.admissions@admin.ox.ac.uk
Web: http://www.ox.ac.uk

Clinical Medical School Offices (graduate admissions)
John Radcliffe Hospital
Headington
Oxford OX3 9DU
Tel: 01865 2700 59/60/80
   01865 221 686 (general medical school offices)
Fax: 01865 270049
Email: graduate.admissions@admin.ox.ac.uk
Web: http://www.medsci.ox.ac.uk

Oxford

Additional application information

Average A-level requirements	• AAA, including chemistry
Average Scottish Higher requirements	• AAAAA and CSYS, Advanced Highers
Graduate entry requirements	• 2:1 or better in a bioscience or chemistry degree
Make-up of interview panel	• Preclinical: one or two college Fellows
	• Clinical: panel of four including clinicians, preclinical teachers, at least one woman
	• Graduate intake: typically one clinician and one college tutor
Months in which interviews are held	• Preclinical: December
	• Clinical: late January early February
	• Graduate intake: December
Proportion of overseas students	• 4% preclinical, 7% clinical
Proportion of mature students	• Up to 2%
Proportion of graduate students	• Up to 2%
Faculty's view of students taking a gap year	• Generally supportive if good reasons but consult individual college admission tutors
Proportion of students taking intercalated degrees	• 100% (the Honours degree is part of the course)
Possibility of direct entrance to clinical phase	• Yes (Honours graduates only) with preclinical qualification undertaken in the UK
Fees for overseas students	• £10 424 pa (preclincial) £19 108 pa (clinical). Non EU students pay college fees of £2000–£4000
Fees for graduates	• See Chapter 6
Ability to transfer to other medical schools	• Yes – this is possible after completing the 3-year preclinical component of the course, but only to other universities (mainly Cambridge and some London medical schools), which run a predominantly non-integrated course
Assistance for elective funding	• Yes – there are a variety of funds available. Each college has its own travel bursaries, as does the medical school itself

Assistance for travel to attachments	• With placements outside Oxford, the medical school will reimburse travel costs in full (where accommodation is provided, this comprises just one return journey per week)
Access and hardship funds	• These are administered mainly through the individual colleges, and are always available, but vary in value and criteria for application
Weekly rent	• £65–£95 (varies with college)
Pint of lager	• From £2.50 upwards!
Cinema	• About £5 – there are good cinemas though, including great arts ones
Nightclub	• Lots to choose from; mostly about £5 entry with cheap drinks. There are always student promotions on

Peninsula (Exeter and Plymouth)

Key facts	Undergraduate
Course length	5 years
Total number of medical undergraduates	302
Applicants in 2003	1027
Interviews given in 2003	756
Places available in 2003	167
Places available in 2004	167
Open days 2004	25 and 26 June,16 June (Plymouth), 22 June (Exeter)
Entrance requirements	AAA + 1AS (370 points)
Mandatory subjects	One science subject
Male:female ratio	–
Is an exam included in the selection process? If yes, what form does this exam take?	No
Qualification gained	BMBS

Note: students are allocated randomly to a campus.

As part of the expansion of medical school places in the UK, the government has sanctioned the opening of several new schools. One of the new institutions is the product of collaboration between the Universities of Exeter and Plymouth, and is called the Peninsula Medical School (PMS). As well as being new in the physical sense, Peninsula is also very new in its approach to medical training. The course is designed to reflect the NHS's increasing emphasis on health services within the community and the less obvious divisions between primary and secondary care. Therefore, the medical school is determined that its students will have a wider understanding of all aspects of patient care. From week 1 of the BMBS course, students will spend time in the community developing their clinical skills – learning from GPs, nurses, and other healthcare professionals as they go about their daily working lives. This practical experience of working as part of a team is seen as crucially important in a modernised health service that aims to put the patient, rather than bureaucracy, at the heart of future strategic planning.

In October 2002, 127 students commenced their BMBS degree. This figure rose to 167 in 2003, and by 2007, the school will be training approximately 800 new doctors. There is no such thing as a typical Peninsula student and there is a high percentage of mature students; previous careers range from scientists to opera singers. This makes for a very good social mix. However, being split over several sites means that you may never get to know other people in your year, who are always on other sites.

Education

At Peninsula, students learn about medical topics and medically related issues in terms of the different stages in the life cycle of a human being. Each stage of human life, from conception to old age, is covered in a 2-week long case unit of which there are 10 in years 1 and 2. In year 1, emphasis is placed on the normal functions of the body, whereas in year 2 the emphasis is on pathology. The lectures, clinical skills, and placements during a case unit aim to supplement the learning objectives for that case unit. For example, during the "Conception" case unit, students research topics such as the menstrual cycle, reproductive system, and fertility, while also visiting family planning clinics on their placements and learning how to carry out appropriate clinical examinations, such as vaginal examinations and listening to the babies' heart in a pregnant patient.

Teaching

PMS is part of a new breed of medical schools in which the medical course is based less on the traditional didactic methods of teaching such as lectures, relying more on problem-based learning (PBL). PBL involves students working in small groups to determine learning objectives, researching these learning objectives, and sharing the information that they obtained in subsequent PBL sessions. Anatomy, cell biology/histology, and medical imaging teaching are incorporated into life science sessions once a week where students work with both life-like as well as live human models to identify important anatomical structures and their clinical significance. Another main part of teaching time is spent in clinical skills, where practical and communication skills are taught. This includes anything from interviewing an actor in the role of an alcoholic patient to practising taking blood.

Assessment

Each student is assessed in four areas throughout the course of Phase 1 (years 1 and 2). The Progress Test is an MCQ exam that the students sit four times each year – this assesses their level of applied medical knowledge (AMK). This exam is not based directly on previous work – rather, it aims to assess progress across the board in all aspects of AMK, and all year groups sit the same paper at the same time. This might mean that students starting the course get very low "marks" but are deemed satisfactory within their year-group, but by year 5 are expected to get very high marks. The students are also assessed in modules for special study units (SSU), clinical skills, and personal and professional development (PPD). Each student must pass all four areas at the end of the year 2 to commence on to Phase 2 of the course (years 3 and 4). In addition, a practical assessment of clinical skills is carried out at the end of years 1 and 2 in the form of an integrated structured clinical examination (ISCE) – known everywhere else as an OSCE. SSU reports are written in the style of a scientific paper and, at the time of writing, are marked on style rather than content in Phase 1. Reflective analyses reports are used to assess the PPD module alongside portfolios of staff "reports" on each student.

Intercalated degrees

Intercalated degrees are still in the developmental stages at the moment and may possibly be available for students after year 4. There is also the possibility that students will be able to decide whether they wish to intercalate a traditional BSc degree programme or a non-traditional BA degree programme into their medical course – both of which will be of 1 year's duration.

Special study modules and electives

Peninsula offers special study units (SSU) from year 1 of the course. During Phase 1 these are mostly short, 2-week placements, providing each student with the opportunity to research medical issues and topics of personal interest ranging from clinical- (eg stroke management) or scientific-based topics (eg psychoneuroimmunology) to topics relating to alternative medicine and community (eg shiatsu, yoga).

The structure of SSUs in Phases 2 and 3 of the course has not yet been established, although it is likely that they will be longer and that reports will be marked on content. Due to the relative infancy of the Peninsula course, electives have not yet been taken. However, it seems most likely they will be at the end of year 4.

Erasmus

It is not yet clear if this will be established as part of the medical course at Peninsula.

Facilities

Library   In Exeter, the medical students have access to the resources available at the postgraduate medical centre library as well as the local Institute of Health Studies library. In Plymouth, students have access to the central university library. This is still developing its medical section. Students also have access to hospital libraries in Exeter, Plymouth, and Truro, and these are often very helpful.

Computers   In both Exeter and Plymouth, Peninsula provides a dedicated IT suite for medical students.

Clinical skills   Peninsula is particularly keen on students developing clinical skills; a 2-hour session forms part of the timetable each week from the first week onwards. Students attend a clinical skills session in a purpose-built clinical skills centre where they practise carrying out core skills, such as basic life support, taking blood, physical examinations, measuring blood pressure. One of the other main themes worked on in clinical skills is development of communication skills; from initiating the consultation to practising patient interviews with actors. These may vary from interviewing a "patient" with a sore tummy to a "patient" with suspected schizophrenia! The actors are remarkably convincing!

Welfare

Student support

As students of the Universities of Exeter and Plymouth, each PMS student has access to all of the student support services available in their locality. This includes the welfare and equal opportunities offices, student counselling centre, student advice centre, education unit, as well as Nightline, the University of Exeter's student support hotline. For students with families, support is also available from the student parent department and family centre.

One of the challenges for all students is moving to Truro as everyone is based there for at least 1 year. This is because, at the current time there is no student provision in Truro. However, the senior staff at Truro are keen to remedy this and are developing support mechanisms.

Accommodation

Accommodation is provided for all year 1 students in Exeter and Plymouth and year 3 students in Truro. The accommodation provided in Exeter is within walking distance of the campus, hospitals, and many of the GP surgeries that students will visit for their placements. It is also conveniently located next to a number of restaurants and banks as well as a chemist and grocery shop that is open until late. Year 1 accommodation in Plymouth is usually in the student halls of residence, which are central to the university and city centre.

Placements

Placements may be anywhere across the South West, and free accommodation may be offered if you are away from your "home" campus.

Sports and social 🏆

City life

Exeter is a city packed with a blend of modern and historical attractions for students. These range from popular nightspots in the city centre and on the waterfront, to the magnificent Exeter Cathedral, surrounded by cobbled alleyways and catacombs. Most of the popular bars, nightclubs, and cinemas are located in the town centre, which is only 10 minutes away from campus by foot. The regular jazz and comedy nights held on the waterfront are not to be missed either.

Plymouth is a *big city* down south. It has an interesting mixture of the traditional Devon appeal (clotted cream teas) and a modern edge. If you love the sea, this is the place for you. Many sailors

Location of clinical placement/name of hospital	Distance away from medical school (miles)	Difficulty getting there on public transport*	Accommodation available
Royal Devon & Exeter	0	+	No
Derriford Hospital	7	++	No
GP placements, Plymouth	0–10	+/+++	No
Treliske Hospital	6	++	Yes
Phase 2 – GP placements	Across South-West England	+++	Yes

*Ease of accessibility: +, set your alarm clock early; ++, long journey; +++, car is a must

and surfers live here. It's also not far from Dartmoor, which provides stunning scenery and the opportunity for fantastic outdoor pursuits.

Plymouth is a budding new university. Within the university, students are housed in a large new building, which is part of a planned development giving new arts space to the university and the city. Plymouth may not have the long-standing academic tradition of some colleges; but it does offer the advantage of exciting development allied with open-mindedness and terrific enthusiasm. If you are interested in research, this is a good place to be.

University life

Plymouth and Exeter provide rather different student experiences. In Plymouth, medical students are integrated into the student population – the halls in year 1 are mixed and many second-year medics live with other non-medic students. By contrast, medical students in Exeter are mainly based on a separate campus from the other Exeter students and are hence less integrated into the wider university. The Medical Societies (MedSoc) on both sites have similar aims and provide similar social events, for example lots of going out, sometimes with charity fundraising, themed evenings, etc. Plymouth MedSoc also has an "academic" arm; organising lectures and study sessions – it is planned to widen this to Exeter in the near future. There is also a development of (less alcoholic) events which involve families; we have a fair number of mature students with children. Another highlight is the MedSoc balls; at the time of writing, Exeter hosts the Christmas ball and Plymouth the Summer ball. Last year both were excellent and well attended.

MedSIN (Medical Students' International Network) groups in Exeter and Plymouth are rapidly growing and have started to attract attention from other student societies and students. MedSIN offers students the opportunity to run and participate in numerous different community projects such as Marrow, Sexpression, and CPR in local schools.

Sports life

Both the main campus and St Luke's campus in Exeter have well-maintained sports halls that include a gym and swimming pool as well as basketball, badminton, and squash courts. The Athletic Union in Exeter has over 40 sports clubs (including seven different kinds of martial arts) ranging from archery to windsurfing. The watersports (subaqua, surfing) are extremely popular as there are regular trips on the weekends to the coast and nearby beaches.

Plymouth University has its own sailing and diving centre, which provides taught courses at a small cost. The number of sports clubs is enormous – and if they don't have what you want, you can set up your own club. Intraschool sports competitions are also being developed. The first two annual football matches (Plymouth versus Exeter) have taken place (with both boys and girls teams) and rugby is planned to follow soon.

> **Fascinating fact:** The "Pilgrim Fathers" set off from Plymouth to Newfoundland on the "Mayflower".

Great things about Peninsula 👍

- Students learn clinical skills from the first week.
- It is only a short drive/train ride to the beach.
- Small year groups so no one is a stranger.
- Compared to the bigger cities, living in Exeter is relatively inexpensive.
- The brand new medical school buildings, with brand new facilities, exclusively available to the medical students, are excellent.

Bad things about Peninsula 👎

- The medical school doesn't have a library yet.
- After years 1 and 2 in either Exeter or Plymouth, students are rotated around various Peninsula Medical School locations in Devon and Cornwall (Exeter, Plymouth, Truro, Barnstaple, Torbay). A downer if you're looking to settle down in one place.
- Peninsula doesn't have an assessment-based learning approach – this may not be good if you are not self-motivated.
- You may never get to meet other students in your year if they move to other campuses at different times from you.
- Students in Exeter don't get to choose their halls of residence in year 1. If a student decides to stay in a hall of residence, effectively he or she has to stay in either Rowancroft Court or Mews as these are the only halls that are based near to the campus and that offer hall agreements for 40 weeks.

Further information

Medical Admissions Office
Peninsula Medical School
ITTC Building
Tamar Science Park
Davy Road
Plymouth PL6 8BX
Tel: 01752 764 261
Fax: 01752 764 226
Email: medadmissions@pms.ac.uk
Web: http://www.pms.ac.uk

Additional application information

Average A-level requirements	• AAA + 1 AS (370 points, preferably including one science and one non-science subject)
Average Scottish Higher requirements	• Minimum 340 points from 5 Highers in both science and non-science subjects or AAB Advanced Highers
Graduate entry requirements	• GAMSAT
Make-up of interview panel	• Three panel members from the following: clinicians, healthcare practitioners, non-clinical academics, lay community
Months in which interviews are held	• November, December, March
Proportion of overseas students	• 0%
Proportion of mature students	• 20% (non-direct school leavers)
Proportion of graduate students	• c 15–20%
Faculty's view of students taking a gap year	• Acceptable
Proportion of students taking intercalated degrees	• New school, no information at present
Possibility of direct entrance to clinical phase	• No
Fees for overseas students	• N/A
Fees for graduates	• See Chapter 6
Ability to transfer to other medical schools	• Possible
Assistance for elective funding	• New school, no information at present
Assistance for travel to attachments	• Available
Access and hardship funds	• Available
Weekly rent	• £65
Pint of lager	• Relatively inexpensive at the Union bar
Cinema	• £3–£4
Nightclub	• £5

Royal Free and University College

Key facts	Undergraduate
Course length	6 years
Total number of medical undergraduates	2800
Applicants in 2003	2340
Interviews given in 2003	994
Places available in 2003	330
Places available in 2004	330
Open days 2004	April
Entrance requirements	AAB + AS
Mandatory subjects	Chemistry plus biology at A or AS-level
Male:female ratio	2:3
Is an exam included in the selection process?	Yes
If yes, what form does this exam take?	BMAT
Qualification gained	MBBS + BSc

The Royal Free and University College London Medical School (RF&UCMS) is the product of the recent merger of two world-class institutions: Royal Free Hospital School of Medicine (Hampstead) and University College London Medical School (Bloomsbury). It is one of the largest medical schools in the UK and lies in an exciting, attractive, and vibrant part of London. Both parent schools have excellent reputations for teaching and research and include a number of world-famous institutions, including the Institute of Child Health (Great Ormond Street), the Institute of Neurology (the National Hospital for Neurology and Neurosurgery), the Institute of Laryngology and Otology, and the Institute of Ophthalmology (Moorfields Eye Hospital). RF&UCMS offers a modern course, attended by some very friendly students and taught by respected academics and clinicians.

Education

The new curriculum started in 2000. It is a 6-year integrated systems-based course, including an intercalated BSc for non-graduates. Clinical experience starts from day one, although the preclinical/clinical divide has not been entirely abandoned.

Teaching

The core curriculum is arranged into three distinct phases. Phase I consists of systems-based learning modules, which cover all basic medical subjects. Phase II (science and medical practice, years 3 and 4) consists of a series of sequential clinical attachments, reflecting and building on the systems-based modules of Phase I. In year 3 there are two half-days of formal teaching (including basic science) each week, and in year 4 there are blocks of formal teaching (again including basic science) between clinical attachments. In Phase III (professional development and year 5), there are clinical attachments in general practice, A&E, and district general hospitals, as well as selective specialist clinical attachments and a period of elective study.

Running throughout these sequential modules for all 5 years of the course there are three vertical modules: mechanisms of drug action/use of medicines; society and the individual; and pathology. There is also a continuous strand of professional development from year 1 through to year 5.

Assessment

Assessment includes MCQs, OSCEs, and oral examinations. It is integrated with a considerable amount of formative assessment and a portfolio of coursework that must be completed to a satisfactory standard in order to permit entry to the end-of-year summative assessments that ultimately determine progression.

Intercalated degrees

All non-graduate students are expected to complete an intercalated BSc. Although the majority of students will intercalate between Phases I and II, some will choose to do so later in the medical degree programme, especially if they wish to pursue a BSc programme designed for students with greater clinical experience. The range of subjects to choose from is impressive and new intercalated BSc course units and degree programmes in 2002 were extended to include medical ethics and law, forensic archaeology, and space physiology and medicine. Information on the intercalated BSc is given to students in year 2.

Special study modules and electives

In addition to the core curriculum, there are special study modules to permit the study of selected aspects in depth. These may be medical or non-medical and can include law, history of medicine, arts, and modern languages. Four must be taken in Phase I, three in Phase II, and two in Phase III. In addition, a period of elective study is taken in the final year and most students choose to spend this abroad. Limited funding is available.

Erasmus

There are currently no opportunities for exchange under the ERASMUS programme, and travel overseas is generally restricted to the elective period, although some people have been known to "sneak off" to Trinidad for their paediatric rotations.

Facilities

Library   There are large medical and clinical science libraries on the Bloomsbury campus, a well-stocked and spacious library on the Hampstead campus, and a new and well-stocked library on the Archway (Whittington Hospital) campus. In addition, the many postgraduate medical institutes associated with UCL have specialist libraries within easy walking distance of Gower Street. The British Museum is a stone's throw away from the Bloomsbury campus as is the Wellcome Institute, the Institute of Neurology, the School of Pharmacy, and the London School of Hygiene and Tropical Medicine.

Computers   There are clusters of networked computers throughout all RF&UCMS campus sites and in many halls of residence. When the rooms are not booked for formal teaching, students have free access on a first-come first-served basis. Most networked computers are Windows PCs, although there are some Apple computers. All students have free internet and email access and free printing resources, as well as a wide variety of networked software. IT skills are assessed at the beginning of the course, and there is a scheme for peer tutoring.

Clinical skills   There are clinical skills laboratories on all three "home" campuses, and in addition to timetabled sessions, students may arrange access at other times. They are all well liked by students, allowing such diverse activities as suturing sponges, cannulating plastic arms, and catheterising plastic penises!

Welfare

Student support

In Phase I, all students are assigned a personal tutor/academic adviser, normally a basic scientist who oversees their personal and academic development and provides pastoral care. In Phases II and III, students are assigned personal tutors who are clinically qualified. In addition, the faculty tutorial team provide regular "walk-in surgeries", and most academic staff in UCL have an open-door policy or clearly advertised hours when they are available to students. UCL has a wide range of welfare, support, and counselling services available to all students.

Student feedback on course quality and teaching is actively sought through questionnaires, faculty education committees, and staff–student consultative committees. Courses will be changed in the light of (valid) student comments. Organisation is generally very good, with comprehensive lecture notes being provided by lecturers as lectures and formal tutorials still form an important part of the new course.

Location of clinical placement/name of hospital	Distance away from medical school (miles)	Difficulty getting there on public transport*	Accommodation available
UCH/Middlesex	0	+	No
Royal Free	0	+	No
Whittington	0	+	No

*Ease of accessibility: +, set your alarm clock early; ++, long journey; +++, car is a must

Aooommodation

Practically all first-year students stay in UCL or University of London halls. Halls are generally acceptable, and a second year in halls is normally available during the BSc or final year. The accommodation office at Senate House offers help and legal advice to London students. To find better-value accommodation, many students choose to travel into central London from places like Finsbury Park and Camden.

The minimum you should expect to pay is £65. However, you will find yourself fighting with the commuters for at least 40 minutes every morning. As a result, most RF&UCMS students pay £80–100 per week to live in zone 2. If you are blessed with wealth then you might be tempted by a shoebox in zone 1, for convenience if not for comfort!

Placements

There are three main campuses, which make up the Royal Free and University College Medical School: the Bloomsbury site (UCH/Middlesex), the Hampstead site (Royal Free), and the Archway site (Whittington). Most teaching in Phase 1 takes place at the Bloomsbury site, except teaching for the Professional Development Spine (PDS), which is split across the three.

Most clinical teaching placements (Phases 2 and 3) are at UCH/Middlesex, Royal Free, and Whittington Hospitals, all of which are in central London and are easily accessible by public transport.

There are numerous district general hospital attachments during years 4 and 5. Many of these are located in the home counties, although some are further afield (Truro, Stoke-on-Trent). For the DGH attachments, accommodation is usually provided, since they are more difficult to get to by public transport. Where accommodation is unavailable, travel costs are reimbursed.

Sports and social ♔

City life

UCL's central London location places students very close to some of the finest theatres, concert halls, and museums in the world. The Royal Free campus has both the cosmopolitan atmosphere of

Hampstead and the green scenery of Hampstead Heath. In nearby Camden there are opportunities to see live music and visit Camden Lock market. The famous areas of Soho and Covent Garden are only a short walk away from the Bloomsbury campus.

University life

Students of the medical school are, like all UCL students, members of University College London Union, and they enjoy all the facilities and services that the Union provides. Medical students form a very large group within the total student population, and their special needs are provided for by medical Student Union Officers on all three sites. As a community, we call ourselves "RUMS" (Royal Free and University College Medical Students).

The family-like community of medical students here is encouraged from day 1, when freshers are given a second-year "parent" to guide them through the first months of medical student life. Throughout the year, the RUMS officers organise various events, including balls, theme nights, and shows, beginning with the 14-day extravaganza of RUMS freshers' fortnight. As well as organising a Rag week and running more than 30 clubs and societies, the RUMS officers also represent medical students to the school on educational and welfare-related issues.

Medical students have their own bar/clubhouse in Huntley Street on the Bloomsbury campus, as well as social and Union facilities at the Royal Free campus. In addition, there is the main UCL Union, with centres on the Bloomsbury campus and in the Windeyer Building (part of the Middlesex Hospital site, a few minutes' walk from Gower Street). The excellent University of London Union (ULU) is directly adjacent to the Bloomsbury campus. This means that there is an unparalleled variety of sports and social facilities available, with opportunities to meet students from other disciplines.

Your motto will become "work hard, play hard" and there is something for every RUMS student to enjoy: we have our own medic societies as well as the hundreds of Union societies to choose from. We also have our traditional medics' "comedy" revue company, which puts on an annual Christmas show for the benefit of the Middlesex Hospital, not to mention our legendary balls, together with the official Union entertainment. All dramatic, musical, and operatic performances are shown in the college's own renowned West End venue on campus, the UCL Bloomsbury.

One of the most anticipated events is Rag week, which is an orgy of money collecting for charity. You will get up at 5 am to shake a tin at a tube station and go to bed at 3 am having exhausted yourself at a party or pub-crawl. This is a massive event in the social calendar that we all look forward to. The societies organise social events ranging from "civilised" dinners to rather less civilised initiations, and put on plays and musical shows alongside gigs and choral performances. Don't forget that at RUMS you are not confined to socialising within the medical school – you also have the varied clubs and societies of UCL to explore.

Sports life

You can play for RUMS in most sports, but you are also entitled to play for the UCL Union and ULU teams if you wish. They all compete in both national and local competitions in most sports. RUMS teams play at UCL's sports ground in Shenley, Hertfordshire. This is a 60-acre site catering for most sports and is the home ground of the UCL Union teams as well. When not in use for such important fixtures some second-rate, semiprofessional team called Watford FC are permitted to train there! UCL has a very strong tradition of water-based sports. We row from the university boathouse in Chiswick. One highlight of the sporting year is the United Hospital Bumps for eights on the Thames. The swimming pool in the basement of John Astor House is available to medical students, as are the weights room, gym, squash courts, and billiards rooms. Somers Town Sports Centre is a new and important venue for UCL sports situated near the Bloomsbury campus. It offers excellent facilities for a number of the RUMS teams, including the basketball, netball, hockey, and football clubs. The Union also provides an impressive gym complex, the Bloomsbury Fitness Centre. Finally, UCL students have full access to ULU facilities and societies and there is a large swimming pool, jacuzzi, and sauna in the nearby Malet Street buildings. Of special interest are the various United Hospital sports clubs in which all members of our students' society are encouraged to participate.

Fascinating fact: The Royal Free Hospital was the first in the country to train women as doctors.

Great things about RF&UCMS

- One of the top-ranking universities in the UK for research in basic medical sciences and clinical medicine, with a school truly integrated into the multifaculty institution of UCL with all the associated benefits in terms of sporting, cultural, and social facilities.
- UCL's central London location places RF&UCMS students very close to some of the finest theatres, concert halls, and museums in the world. The Royal Free campus has both the cosmopolitan atmosphere of Hampstead and the green scenery of Hampstead Heath.
- Plenty of opportunity to mix socially and academically with non-medics at a multifaculty university with many BSc opportunities.
- A major centre of biomedical research, with opportunities to work alongside world leaders in research at a school renowned for its teaching system, with plenty of small-group tutorials, a superbly equipped dissection suite and new teaching and learning facilities.
- RF&UCMS medics are members of their own Union, the UCL Union, and the University of London Union, so there is no shortage of student activity even though the opportunities of central London are on your doorstep.

Bad things about RF&UCMS

- Central London can be a little daunting at first if you're not used to living in a big city; and crossing Euston Road every day can't be good for your health with its combination of pollution and dangerous drivers!
- The need to travel around London to get to different campuses – Bloomsbury (UCH), Archway (Whittington), and Hampstead (Royal Free) – and the fact that you probably won't be able to avoid a 20-minute tube journey into college after you leave halls, unless you're lucky or rich!
- Living in London is only as expensive as you make it, but the rent is ridiculous. Expect to pay £100 a week. Visible signs of poverty can be depressing.

- In a class of 330, it can be easy to be isolated and not meet all of your fellow students, especially in the early years. As UCL is a 16 000-strong college you can feel like a very small fish in a very large pond when you first arrive.
- Tough retake policy; for example in year 1 students must pass a further three papers with an overall pass of 50%, rather than resitting the one failed paper as with many other medical schools.

Further information

Faculty Tutor
Faculty of Life Sciences
University College London
London WC1E 6BT
Tel: 020 7679 5467/5493
Fax: 020 7679 5494
Email: medicaladmissions@ucl.ac.uk
Web: http://www.ucl.ac.uk/medical school

Students' Union: Medical Students' and Sites' Officer
25 Gordon Street
London WC1H 0AY
Tel: 020 7679 7949
Email: mss.officer@ucl.ac.uk
Web: http://www.uclu.org.uk

Additional application information

Average A-level requirements	• AAB, to include chemistry, plus biology at A or AS-level. Plus a pass in a fourth AS-level. GCSE maths and English
Average Scottish Higher requirements	• Three Advanced Highers at AAB
Graduate entry requirements	• 2:1 degree + BBC. Graduates and non-graduates follow the same course
Make-up of interview panel	• Three, comprising clinician, scientist and one other
Months in which interviews are held	• November–March (January for graduates)
Proportion of overseas students	• 8%
Proportion of mature students	• No information
Proportion of graduate students	• 14%
Faculty's view of students taking a gap year	• Positive
Proportion of students taking intercalated degrees	• 100% (excluding graduates)
Possibility of direct entrance to clinical phase	• Usually Oxbridge only
Fees for overseas students	• £19 110
Fees for graduates	• See Chapter 6
Ability to transfer to other medical schools	• Not normally, only in extenuating circumstances
Assistance for elective funding	• Not normally available from the college – apply to outside trusts
Assistance for travel to attachments	• Travel outside zone 2 is refunded. If accommodation is provided only one return journey is paid for
Access and hardship funds	• UCL has a large Access Fund available to all its students throughout the year. However there are 10 000 undergraduates at UCL, so it is advisable to get applications in early
Weekly rent	• £65–£100
Pint of lager	• 99p on Mondays! £1.65 on other week nights
Cinema	• £5 upwards in the city. (£2 at UCL Union Film Society for slightly older films)
Nightclub	• £5–£20 depending on club and night

St Andrew's

Key facts	Undergraduate
Course length	6 years (3 years at Manchester/Keele/Preston)
Total number of medical undergraduates	350
Applicants in 2003	557
Interviews given in 2003	50
Places available in 2003	125
Places available in 2004	125
Open days 2004	14, 21, 28, April
Entrance requirements	ABB
Mandatory subjects	Chemistry + another science
Male:female ratio	40:60
Is an exam included in the selection process? If yes, what form does this exam take?	No
Qualification gained	BMedSci

Established in the 15th century, St Andrew's is the oldest university in Scotland. It is set in a small picturesque town on the east coast of Fife. The course lasts for 3 years, during which the importance of the traditional preclinical subjects is emphasised. After this, the vast majority of students head south for Manchester, where they complete their clinical studies (a further 3 years). The uniqueness of such a course provides a great opportunity for students to experience studying both in an ancient university town and in a big vibrant city. The faculty is small and students socialise with medics and non-medics alike.

Education

St Andrew's is the oldest university in Scotland, which explains the traditions and customs that surround being a student here. The course is quite traditional, being departmentalised rather than integrated, but it is frequently reviewed and improved to suit the needs of a modern doctor in training. The first 2 years are spent learning anatomy, physiology, cellular and molecular medicine, and behavioural sciences. A first-aid course is also completed in year 1. Second-year students choose an SSM in the second semester, which is usually in the form of a project, as well as completing a course called Assessing Medical Evidence, covering skills in numeracy, critical thinking, experimental design, and evidence-based medicine. Year 3 is spent studying microbiology, pharmacology, pathology, public health, applied medical science, and behavioural sciences. The course still has a very traditional preclinical feel and there is little patient contact, although clinical relevance is always emphasised. The small class size for tutorials and dissection gives a great opportunity to develop good relationships between students and with staff.

Students graduate in medical sciences and then progress to a clinical school for a further 3 years before graduating as a doctor. There is a guaranteed place at Manchester and the vast majority go there, although a small number are given places at Preston or Keele. Students are at liberty to apply to another school for their clinical studies if they so wish. Some aspects of the preclinical course mimic the problem-based learning approach in operation at Manchester, and integration between the two schools has improved greatly over the last few years. One of the benefits of the course structure at St Andrew's is that students leave here with a degree whether or not they continue medical studies.

Teaching

Teaching is by lectures, tutorials, and practicals, with some tutorials using computer-based teaching. Anatomy is taught using cadavers, which the students dissect.

Assessment

Exams are varied and often include a mixture of MCQs, short-answer questions, essays, case studies, and vivas. Mid-terms and practical work done throughout the year contribute a small amount towards the end of year mark.

Intercalated degrees

An intercalated year is possible at the end of year 3 for those who wish to convert their BSc into an Honours degree. Approximately 20% stay on for this additional year, including most of those who wish to apply to medical schools other than Manchester for their clinical studies.

Special study modules and electives

As the St Andrew's course is purely preclinical, electives are not taken until students transfer to a clinical school. However, a special study module in year 2 provides students with the opportunity to study such subjects as philosophy, ethics, and counselling, as well as more scientific topics such as gastrointestinal imaging and wound healing.

Erasmus

Currently there are no opportunities for medical science students at St Andrew's to take part in the ERASMUS scheme.

Facilities

Library   Opening hours are: Monday to Thursday 9 am–10 pm, Friday to Saturday 9 am–6 pm, and Sunday 1 pm–7 pm. A reasonable range of books is available, but many students buy the core texts because of the restricted availability of some titles. Opening hours are increased during exam periods.

Computers   There are several computer rooms available and halls of residence have computer facilities. The university runs a 24-hour service in computer laboratories scattered around town, including the medical building.

Clinical skills   Access to the laboratory is good and the staff are helpful. Skills such as examining x rays, taking blood, taking blood pressure, and neurological examination of patients are incorporated into the course.

Welfare

Student support

This is an area of major strength at St Andrew's. In such a small town the medics are well integrated into the university, and students have the chance to get to know everyone at the school and make friends outside the faculty. The Dean and faculty staff are very supportive, and tend to get to know everyone by name quite quickly. The Students' Union provides welfare and counselling services, including a "Nightline" service for stressed students. The locals are mostly student friendly, if only because the university is the biggest local employer and students almost outnumber the locals. However, when the revelry surrounding some of the ancient traditions still upheld by the university gets a bit over the top, town and gown relations can become a little strained.

Accommodation

All students can spend their first year in university accommodation (halls and flats), and there are some rooms available for further years. Rooms are often shared and the standard of flats is generally good. Some halls are better than others, but none is bad. Other privately owned accommodation is available, over which the university has no control, and rents average £55–£80 a week. Parking is difficult if you want to live in the town centre. There is a housing office at the university, which can help you find places.

Placements

The medical school consists mainly of the Bute Medical Building, referred to by students as "The Bute". Some other buildings in St Andrew's may be used, but they are all within walking distance of each other. St Andrew's is very small for a university town, so there is no problem getting around.

Students are attached to a local GP clinic in year 2 for only a day, and there are two hospital visits as part of the course in year 3.

Location of clinical placement/name of hospital	Distance away from medical school (miles)	Difficulty getting there on public transport*
St Andrew's Health Centre	0.5	+

*Ease of accessibility: +, set your alarm clock early; ++, long journey; +++, car is a must

Patient contact in St Andrew's is virtually non-existent: it is a true preclinical course. (For clinical placements, see the Manchester chapter.)

Sports and social 🏆

City life

St Andrew's is a beautiful coastal town with a population of less than 20 000, and is famed for its golf course. Being the oldest of Scotland's four ancient universities, it has more than its fair share of traditions and some of the oldest student societies. The students all live very near the centre of town, so it is never far to walk to meet a friend. There is a very good atmosphere among the students, with plenty of chances to mix with medics and non-medics, and enough things going on in the town, at the Union, and with the societies to keep you as busy as you want to be. Tourists and golf followers can make the town bustle a bit too much at times, but you can go celebrity spotting with some success.

The town has easily enough pubs, restaurants, and cafés to keep most people happy, but clubbers and shopaholics will have to travel to Edinburgh or Dundee for some real action. Outdoor types have easy access to the Grampian Mountains, and the nearby sea and beaches can be good fun. There is no railway station at St Andrew's, the nearest being Leuchars, which has regular bus services, or taxis, which cost about £8.

University life

The Union is good – especially for freshers getting to know the place – and alcohol is reasonably cheap, but the club scene is lacking, with very few bands or comedians. There are coaches weekly to nightclubs in Dundee, 30 minutes away, which offer clubbers the chance to visit some of the busiest clubs in Scotland. The price for these buses is £5, which includes entrance to the club and a bus back to St Andrew's. MedSoc (called "The Bute") has good socials, including a famed ball as well as a raucous revue. MedSoc also has a great new website (http://www.butemedics.co.uk).

There are many different types of societies, from the very sensible to the downright silly. Social life tends to focus around balls and events run by these societies. There is normally something to do each week.

Sports life

Most sports are supported, especially hockey and rugby, and there is a medics' competition every year called the "Hypertrophy". Medical school teams do not play every week, and keen players often get involved with their hall teams or the main university clubs. Interhall competitions are also popular. The facilities have been improved in recent years, such as the gym and athletics union. There is no university swimming pool. It is, of course, golf heaven, with the Royal and Ancient offering excellent deals for students. Membership is around £100 a year, which includes the Old Course.

Fascinating fact: Approximately one-third of St Andrew's population are students.

Great things about St Andrew's

- Small year group and good integration with non-medics.
- Excellent integration between medics in all 3 years.
- Numerous social activities organised by the medical society.
- St Andrew's has a great pub and coffee shop culture.
- Golf – dirt-cheap membership on the best courses in Scotland.

Bad things about St Andrew's

- Limited patient contact and low clinical content to course work.
- No nightclubs, if you discount the Union.
- Not many shops – you will probably shop in your home town or travel to Dundee (a 30-minute bus ride away).
- It can get a bit cold at times.
- Relatively small student numbers can make it difficult to "get away from it all".

Further information

Admissions Office
79 North Street
St Andrews
Fife KY16 9AJ
Tel: 01334 462 150 (schools liaison service)
Tel: 01334 476 161 (switchboard)
Fax: 01334 463 388
Email: admissions@st-andrews.ac.uk
Web: http://www.st-andrews.ac.uk

Additional application information

Average A-level requirements	• ABB at one sitting, including chemistry and one other science
Average Scottish Higher requirements	• AAABB, including chemistry and one other science
Graduate entry requirements	• 2:1 in a science-related degree
Make-up of interview panel	• Three staff usually including admissions tutor, clinician, lecturer, of both genders
Months in which interviews are held	• November–January
Proportion of overseas students	• 20%
Proportion of mature students	• 4%
Proportion of graduate students	• 4%
Faculty's view of students taking a gap year	• Positive
Proportion of students taking intercalated degrees	• 10%
Possibility of direct entrance to clinical phase	• No
Fees for overseas students	• £13 000
Fees for graduates	• See Chapter 6
Ability to transfer to other medical schools	• Guaranteed transfer to Manchester/Preston/Keele for clinical training. Although you can apply to any university for clinical training
Assistance for elective funding	• N/A
Assistance for travel to attachments	• N/A
Access and hardship funds	• Financial department supplies a means tested bursary – several different ones available
Weekly rent	• £55–£80
Pint of lager	• £1.50 at the Union
Cinema	• £3.65
Nightclub	• £3 at Union nightclub

St George's

Key facts	Premedical	Undergraduate	Graduate
Course length	6 years	5/6 years	4 years
Total number of medical undergraduates	16	995	140
Applicants in 2003	45	1600	1500
Interviews given in 2003	25	700	290
Places available in 2003	20	187	70
Places available in 2004	20	187	70
Open days 2004		Last Wednesday of every month at 2 pm (except July and December)	April, June, July, September
Entrance requirements	Some post 16 qualifications or significant career progression	AABB	2:2 degree in any discipline
Mandatory subjects	GCSE English, maths, and science	Chemistry and biology (at least one to A-level)	None
Male:female ratio	1:1	2:3	3:2
Is an exam included in the selection process? If yes, what form does this exam take?	No	No	Yes, GAMSAT
Qualification gained	MBBS	MBBS	MBBS

St George's Hospital Medical School (SGHMS) is located in the heart of Tooting, in south London, 5 minutes' walk from Tooting Broadway Underground station. It genuinely is a very welcoming school, with plenty of atmosphere and a wide variety of clinical experience available. St George's Hospital itself is one of the largest teaching hospitals in Europe, situated in a heavily populated part of London with pressing health needs. It offers two medical degree programmes: an established 5-year course and a 4-year graduate-entry programme. As well as medics, there are nursing, midwifery, physiotherapy, radiography, and biomedical science students at St George's, all of whom mix well with staff to create a strong feeling of community within the hospital. It is this, in particular, that makes SGHMS a great place to study. Most will thoroughly enjoy the atmosphere but, at the very least, all will appreciate it.

Education

The standard course lasts 5 years, with clinical experience starting with visits to GP surgeries in year 1. Since 1996 all new medical students have undertaken the special study modules (SSMs), the aim of which is to allow students to study, in depth, areas of particular interest to them.

Teaching

Year 1 begins with the common foundation module, during which much of the teaching is shared by all the first-year healthcare courses (nurses, physiotherapists, radiographers, biomedical degree students, etc). The rest of the medics' teaching is then divided into two core cycles. In core cycle 1 (years 1 and 2) students study systems modules, integrated with some clinical experience, and undertake two SSMs. In core cycle 2 (years 3–5) students get general clinical experience in hospitals, GP surgeries, etc, covering a wide range of medical and surgical areas. Structured teaching is provided at all clinical attachments, in addition to ongoing lecture programmes at St George's. Students also complete three more SSMs in core cycle 2, the last of which is the elective.

Assessment

Exams take place every term for the first 2 years, and term exams contribute to the end-of-year synoptic exams. These must be passed to progress to the next year. At the end of year 3 students take an exam that accounts for 20% of the final MBBS qualification. Written finals come at the end of year 4 and the elective and clinical finals take place in year 5. Written exams include MCQs (multiple-choice questions), which are negatively marked, EMIS (extended matching items which are essentially long lists from which the correct answer must be chosen), short-answer questions, and, in major exams, essays. Practical skills are assessed with OSPEs or "spotters" which are predominantly anatomy-based and OSCEs, which test clinical skills using actors as patients.

Intercalated degrees

An intercalated BSc can be taken after years 2, 3, or 4. The later the degree is taken the more clinical in nature it can be. Study can be at St George's Hospital or other London colleges/medical schools (or further afield if you so desire) and there is a wide range of courses available. Choices are not restricted to medical or science subjects.

Special study modules and electives

SSMs provide an excellent opportunity to study an area that is of specialist interest. The first two (studied in year 2) must be undertaken at St George's, but from then on the choice is very open. They can even be studied abroad if so desired and this option is particularly popular for the fifth SSM – a two-month elective. Most St George's students follow the pattern of taking the first three at St George's and using the fourth as a "mini elective" before the main elective.

Erasmus

The IFMSA exchange scheme has recently been introduced to St George's. It is a system that allows medical students from across the world to literally swap places for a few weeks. The exchanges scheme is huge and involves over 100 countries, so possibilities are immense.

Facilities

Library At the time of printing, the library is undergoing a multi-million pound refurbishment. Library facilities are extensive, with about 40 000 books, 800 journals on current subscription, and access to a further 77 000 journals. Other facilities include interlibrary loans, photocopying, a large history and archive collection, and an audiovisual room with a large variety of video material.

Computers There is an excellent range of computing facilities available, with networked database, CD-ROM, ZIP and interactive media. The small size of the medical school ensures that one can usually find a computer without queuing. The library has a Unicorn catalogue for public access, over 100 workstations for network access, Word for Windows, Excel, and scanning facilities. There is also a large 24-hour access computer room in the medical school with about 30 terminals and printing facilities. A computer room with eight computer stations is at the halls of residence.

Clinical skills These facilities have been greatly improved in recent years, with an incredible range of realistic models for students to practise on before being faced with real patients. The rooms housing these resources are open 9 am–5 pm Monday to Friday, so students can walk in any time they have a free moment. In addition, the clinical skills facilitator is usually on hand to offer guidance on technique. It is a very valuable resource, which students are encouraged to take advantage of.

Welfare

Student support

Students at St George's tend to be very friendly and easy-going by nature. There is a strong school spirit and students are supportive of each other. All freshers are assigned a "mother" or "father" student to look after them in year 1. There is normally no problem in borrowing lecture notes and getting useful advice. The school has counselling services on-site, and students can use all ULU (University of London Union) facilities.

Accommodation

All first-year students are guaranteed a place in halls but students from all years can apply for a place. The main accommodation costs only £57.50 a week, which represents superb value. It is self-catered and about 10 minutes from the medical school; however, rooms are a bit on the small side, and baths, toilets, and kitchen facilities may have to be shared between six and eight people. Catered accommodation is also available, the same distance from the medical school but costing £95 per week. However, the rooms are significantly bigger and bathroom/kitchen facilities are only shared between three or four. It is also an intercollegiate hall so students from a number of London colleges are able to mix easily.

Tooting itself is filled with eager landlords waiting to accommodate local medical students, and rents in the area are more favourable than in many other parts of London. The average per week is about £70.

Placements

The medical school is part of the main teaching hospital but occupies its own distinct area. There are six floors containing the library, computer rooms, teaching theatres, clinical laboratories, School Club, NatWest Bank, school shop, and offices.

The School Club is the equivalent of a Students' Union. This comprises the student bar, student union offices, a coffee shop, school bookshop, games room, music room, and snooker room. Many students and staff go there to relax for lunch and coffee breaks, and many of the extracurricular activities are held there.

From year 3, students are placed at a variety of different other hospitals for specialty training. Much of the training (normally about three-quarters) will take place at St George's. There is usually a choice of where you go, travel expenses are reimbursed, and accommodation is free. Travel to hospitals other than St George's does not usually take more than 30 minutes to 1 hour by public transport. The distance to attachments increases in the final year, as you reach the end of your training. Many attachments can be an hour or so by public transport, with the furthest being Darlington in the north of the country. However, you are able to choose where you do these attachments, so you are not stuck somewhere where you don't want to be.

Location of clinical placement/name of hospital	Distance away from medical school (miles)	Difficulty getting there on public transport*
Bolingbroke	2	+
Springfield	0	–
St Helier's	4.5	++
Kingston	6.5	+
Epsom	10	+++

*Ease of accessibility: +, set your alarm clock early; ++, long journey; +++, car is a must

Sports and social 🏆

University life

St George's bar is one of the biggest and cheapest in the country, and is the scene of many a great night for many medical students. Discos and club nights are on alternate Friday nights, comedy nights and bands are well attended, and much fun is had by all. There is a wide-screen TV with satellite, films, and the main football and international rugby matches, etc are regularly screened. There is a colossal range of societies and clubs to join, from all the conventional sporting ones like rugby and cricket to a parachuting club and a hill-walking society. There are various religious societies, the orchestra and musical societies, also a debating society – the list is endless. The School Club is very supportive of new clubs.

First and foremost, St George's is now the only freestanding medical school in the UK. The only other students around the place are in the caring professions or professions allied to medicine. There is a great feeling of camaraderie in the college: you will get to know most people in your year and many others. There is much mixing between year groups and with students of the other disciplines, which can be an immense benefit whenever you have questions about the course, etc. This is partly because there are so many social events organised by the Students' Union. The medical school itself encourages students and staff to take as positive an attitude to their extracurricular interests as it does to studying.

Sports life

For the major outdoor sports, St George's uses its own sports ground at Cobham, which is in Surrey. This is about half an hour by coach (provided by the medical school). The rowing teams use the Boat House at Chiswick, where many other London colleges row. At the hospital itself, is the Rob Lowe Sports Centre, which has six squash courts and three general fitness rooms with exercise bikes, treadmills, rowing machines, and step machines. There is also a weights room and a large sports hall for team sports, such as five-a-side football, and basketball. There are regular circuit training and aerobic lessons.

Fascinating fact: St George's Hospital Medical School boasts the longest student bar in the country!

Great things about St George's 👍

- It is a small, close-knit community, with many easy-going, fun-loving people as company, and friendly staff and tutors ready to help you along the way.
- The bar – now newly refurbished and the "best thing since sliced bread", according to the first-years. Definitely the heart and soul of the medical school, and with ridiculously cheap beer to boot!
- Location, location, location! The medical school is one of the biggest teaching hospitals in Europe, giving easy access to loads of weird and wonderful pathologies.

- If you do have to travel to a peripheral site, expenses are reimbursed and accommodation provided.
- Freshers' fortnight – yes, that's right, St George's offers 2 weeks of continuous freshers' events, from the principal's boat party to a three-legged pub-crawl, to numerous random fancy dress discos and the Wimbledon pram race.

Bad things about St George's

- Although you are at a London medical school, St George's cannot pretend it is in central London. Tooting to Leicester Square is about 25 minutes on the tube and 30 minutes on the night bus.
- Lack of students studying anything apart from health sciences can limit the conversation a bit, to say the least!
- Parking at or near the hospital can be difficult and expensive.
- St George's does not have the capacity to offer an intercalated BSc to all its students, although most of those who do want to pursue this course of study usually manage it.
- The hospital canteen food can leave a lot to be desired!

Further information

St George's Hospital Medical School
Cranmer Terrace
London SW17 ORE
Tel: 0208 672 9944
Fax: 0208 725 2734
Email: adm-med@sghms.ac.uk
Web: http://www.sghms.ac.uk

Additional application information

Average A-level requirements	• AAB plus B at AS-level. Chemistry and biology (at least one to A-level)
Average Scottish Higher requirements	• Not accepted
Graduate entry requirements	• 2:2 degree in any discipline
Make-up of interview panel	• Usually three to four members comprising academic staff and senior student
Months in which interviews are held	• November–March (undergraduate course)
	• March (graduate course) January–March (premedical course)
Proportion of overseas students	• 7.5%
Proportion of mature students	• 30%
Proportion of graduate students	• 25%
Faculty's view of students taking a gap year	• Encouraged
Proportion of students taking intercalated degrees	• 25%
Possibility of direct entrance to clinical phase	• No
Fees for overseas students	• £12 475 pa (years 1, 2); £21 875 pa (years 3,4,5)
Fees for graduates	• See Chapter 6
Ability to transfer to other medical schools	• Yes – for clinical years (3, 4, 5)
Assistance for elective funding	• Some but limited. Good resources and help with applications to other funding bodies available
Assistance for travel to attachments	• No, generally attachments are not too far so public transport predominates
Access and hardship funds	• Hardship funds available on request
Weekly rent	• Halls – £57.50 self-catered, £95 catered. Average house/apartment rental in Tooting is £70
Pint of lager	• £1.35
Cinema	• £5 (in Wimbledon)
Nightclub	• George's events are almost always between £2.50–£4

Sheffield

Key facts	Premedical	Undergraduate
Course length	6 years	5 years
Total number of medical undergraduates	19	1150
Applicants in 2003	220	2600
Interviews given in 2003	47	950
Places available in 2003	15	238
Places available in 2004	15	238
Open days 2004	June, July, August, September	
Entrance requirements	ABB	ABB
Mandatory subjects	Non science	Chemistry + another science
Male:female ratio	1:0.72	1:1.7
Is an exam included in the selection process? If yes, what form does this exam take?	No	No
Qualification gained	MBChB	

Sheffield is a city built – like Rome – on seven hills, and is almost, but not quite, as scenic! The university has a very large student population (45 000+) and Sheffield is reputedly one of the best student cities in Britain (see *The Virgin Alternative Guide to British Universities*), and that includes the big place down south. It was awarded the title of UK University of the Year for 2001. The majority of students live and work in the scenic or, in other words, hilly parts of town, but there is a wide variety of areas to choose from. The medical school attracts students from all walks of life and there is a good mixture of backgrounds. The medical course in Sheffield is clinically led and gives students opportunities to start developing their clinical skills from the very start. The two main themes that run throughout the course, clinical competences and medical sciences are linked together by integrated learning activities where students work in teams, and later in the course by themselves, to solve clinical problems. There tends to be one set of exams at the end of each year, and some project work is undertaken in groups throughout the year.

Education

The course is divided into six phases. Phases Ia and Ib are essentially years 1 and 2. Phase II lasts for only 6 months and involves an introduction to clinical medicine. This phase is not examined by written papers but finishes with a set of objective structured clinical exams (or OSCEs) in January. Phases IIIa and IIIb follow this and last two years. Phase IIIa is assessed with both OSCEs and written exams. At the end of Phase IIIb you sit your final written papers for the MBChB. Phase IV starts with 6 months of purely clinical work, and the final OSCEs for the MBChB are taken in the summer.

The clinical course has been redesigned to increase the number of ward attachments, but the time spent on each attachment has had to shorten. These changes have given students a broader range of experience and teaching.

Teaching

The emphasis at Sheffield is on teaching broad concepts rather than detailed facts. This relies on the students' desire to look things up for themselves, and the university hopes to produce doctors who are committed to lifelong learning. There is a lot of anatomy dissection, with plenty of opportunity to get "hands-on" experience, as well as practicals in physiology and biochemistry. Animals are not used in the laboratory, although animal products are. The number of lectures has been reduced to allow time for small-group project work and self-directed learning. Clinical years consist mostly of ward-based attachments, interspersed with lecture blocks and tutorials.

Assessment

Assessment of preclinical students is mainly by end-of-year exams, which comprise written multiple-choice papers and practical spotter exams. The practical exam consists of dissection specimens to test anatomy, physiology, and biochemistry, but there is also continuous assessment through projects and practical write-ups. Additionally, there are brief anonymous tests at the end of each module, which are used as a means to monitor your own progress – otherwise known as formative assessment. In the clinical years, OSCEs are added as well as written papers, and are used to examine clinical skills.

Intercalated degrees

The option of spending an extra year studying for a Bachelor of Medical Science (BMedSci) is open to anyone who has passed all preclinical exams. Funding is available for most places, which are generally research and/or laboratory-based. There is little competition for places and students can "design" their own degree. The faculty publishes a list of projects open to BMedSci students, and staff tend to be very keen to recruit students.

Erasmus

There is no opportunity to participate in an Erasmus programme in Sheffield although students can travel abroad for their elective.

Special study modules and electives

There is one 7-week elective period during year 4. Attachments (if approved by faculty) are usually completed abroad and sufficient help with funding is available from a variety of sources. In addition all clinical students get the opportunity to take special study modules (SSMs) in a subject of personal interest, either chosen from a list available from the medical school or one designed by the student themselves.

Facilities

Library   Libraries are sited around the university and in all hospitals used for teaching. The two main medical libraries have been refurbished and have on-site computer access, including access to the internet and MedLine. Core texts and places to sit are increasing, but be prepared to fight for them at exam time. Opening hours are reasonable, but are limited during weekends.

Computers   There are widespread computer facilities throughout the university and in the Royal Hallamshire Hospital, but be prepared to wait at peak times. One site is open 24 hours. Software provided includes email, internet access, and an increasing number of computer-assisted learning packages which students are encouraged to use.

Clinical skills   There are two new laboratories, one at the Northern General and one at the Royal Hallamshire. The centres provide teaching and assessment in a wide range of practical clinical skills associated with professional duties. The layout of the centre's facilities are designed to encourage self-directed learning with many of the practice rooms simulating a ward environment.

Welfare

Student support

First-year students are eased into the course gently, and there are usually plenty of people around to help with any problems. Most lecturers are willing to help solve academic problems, and the Undergraduate Dean is very approachable. Each student is allocated a tutor as part of a social mentoring group to help with any problems and offer advice. The Students' Union and the university have counsellors and welfare support systems in place and a "buddy scheme" exists, whereby a couple of medical students in year 2 act as "academic parents" for a couple of students in the year below. The point of this is not, as it may at first seem, to be an extension of the nanny state! Instead, it serves to provide a source of information, help, and so on for first-years in case they are unwilling to approach academic staff.

Accommodation

All first-years are guaranteed university-owned accommodation, either in a catered hall of residence or in self-catering accommodation. The standard is good; a major plus being that it is all within easy walking distance of university and in the better part of town. Most (but not all) students move into the private rented sector for their second year. Plenty of housing is available, mostly on 12-month contracts.

Placements

The medical school is based at the Royal Hallamshire Hospital, which is situated adjacent to the main university campus. Preclinical teaching takes place mainly at the medical school, the biomedical

Location of clinical placement/name of hospital	Distance away from medical school (miles)	Difficulty getting there on public transport*	Accommodation available
Royal Hallamshire	0.5	+	No
Rotherham	15	++	Yes
Chesterfield	15	++	No
Doncaster	31	++	Yes
Grimsby	47	+++	Yes

*Ease of accessibility: +, set your alarm clock early; ++, long journey; +++, car is a must

sciences building, and the auditorium within the university Union. The clinical years are taught on the wards of the various Sheffield and peripheral district general hospitals. Lecture blocks for the whole year group are held in the medical school and the excellent Union cinema (!), but smaller groups attend the Northern General Hospital Education Centre. This provides much better teaching facilities, but is situated on the other side of town (20 minutes' drive from the university).

There are five hospitals in the centre of Sheffield, including the two extremely large teaching hospitals – the Northern General and the Royal Hallamshire – and the Sheffield Children's Hospital. The other two are the Weston Park Hospital, specifically for cancer patients, and the newly built Jessops Wing for women at the Royal Hallamshire.

Throughout the clinical phase, there are peripheral attachments in hospitals throughout South Yorkshire and Humberside (up to 50 miles away). There is also a 7-week attachment at a GP practice in or around Sheffield, to which students commute. First-year students shadow a patient suffering from a chronic illness, to assess the impact of disease on daily living. This is known as the community attachment scheme (CAS), and takes a different approach to most of the medical course because of its emphasis on the social effects of disease, rather than how to treat it. Clinical skills, such as history-taking from actual patients, are included from the first term onwards and the intensive clinical experience (ICE) is a new and unique feature of year 1. It follows the Christmas vacation and is a 3-week block enabling early patient contact by the shadowing of doctors, nurses, and social services staff in separate 1-week blocks.

Sports and social 🏆

City life

Sheffield city centre is compact and not terribly well formed, but has a good collection of small shops and restaurants, and Division Street has lots of chic student shops and many bars. Eccleshall Road also boasts many cafés and shops and is situated in the more scenic part of Sheffield, not far from the centre. (Real shopaholics go to the huge purpose-built out-of-town Meadowhall Centre, accessible by bus, train, and tram, which has every high-street store you could wish for). There is an ever-increasing number of new nightclubs, café-bars, and live music venues in Sheffield. As there are many clubs, there is a student night nearly every day of the week, with cheap entry, drinks promotions, and a free bus to and from the venue. There are two theatres and five cinemas within reasonable distance that all have student discounts for those after a bit of culture: the UGC cinema contains the biggest screen in Europe, appropriately called "The Full Monty".

The crowning glory of Sheffield is the Peak District. This attracts many active outdoor types (especially climbers) to the university, as well as those who like to relax over a pint in a nice country pub. Just 10 minutes' drive from the university you can walk, cycle, climb, admire the stunning scenery, and forget all about the pressures of medicine. The locals are generally cheery and it is very easy to quickly settle in Sheffield.

University life

The Medical Society organises regular social events: the annual November ball (be prepared to save up for it), and the medics' revue are particularly well supported, as well as the annual fancy dress three-legged pub crawl and loads of lectures involving free pizza. If you would rather bypass medics after working hours, there are clubs for every taste and style, including Gatecrasher, Republic, Poo Na Na, Kingdom, National Centre for Popular Music, The Leadmill, and the ever-popular NY Sushi. The Students' Union organises cheap and cheerful events every night of the week, including "Pop Tarts". There is a huge variety of clubs and societies available to join: anyone fancy the Warhammer Assassins' Guild, or Star Trek the Whistling Society? Those interested in the more altruistic side to medicine can join the Marrow Appeal set up by medical students, or the Medical Students' International Network (MedSIN), which are both active in Sheffield. In addition, people from all religious denominations are catered for through their respective religious societies. In particular, within the medical school and the Students' Union there are Muslim prayer rooms.

Sports life

The city of Sheffield has inherited a large range of excellent sports facilities after hosting the World Student Games, including the Olympic swimming pool at Pondsforge and Don Valley athletics stadium. Recently a new state of the art gym, swimming pool, and sports centre has been built on campus with all the latest equipment, but unfortunately, the prices are a little steep. All sports are well catered for, but the dry ski slope, indoor climbing wall, and a new ice rink are particular attractions. The medical school has numerous sports teams, with the rugby, football, and hockey clubs all being particularly active.

Fascinating fact: Sir Hans Adolf Krebs taught as leading Professor in pathology between 1935 and 1954 in Sheffield, where he discovered a complicated series of reactions in the body involving the oxidative metabolism of pyruvic acid – he is the founder of "The Krebs cycle", which we all know and love.

Great things about Sheffield 👍

- The course allows individuals to learn at their own pace. Lecturers are very accessible and are usually happy to help with any problems.
- There are still dissection and hands-on practicals instead of prosections.
- There are endless clubs for all music tastes, bars and coffee shops for the trendsetters, and just about every type of entertainment under the sun.
- Student accommodation is in the nicer parts of town, within easy (and safe) walking distance of the university and all local amenities.
- Sheffield medics are down to earth and represent a wide cross-section of society. Medical students are part of the university as a whole, and not just the medical school.

Bad things about Sheffield 👎

- Students complain of poor course organisation, and lack of up-to-date information on the continually changing curriculum.
- Self-directed learning is hard if you are a poor self-motivator and leave things to the last minute; with formal assessment only at the end of the year, it is easy to fall behind.
- According to the consultants, they do not teach anatomy like they used to...or physiology, or biochemistry, etc.
- Some of the peripheral attachments are slightly less than glamorous towns – Hull, Grimsby, Rotherham, Scunthorpe, Barnsley, etc.
- Hills – good practice if you're training for Everest.

Further information

Medical School
University of Sheffield
Beech Hill Road
Sheffield S10 2RX
Tel: 0114 271 3349 (medical school reception)
       0114 271 3727 (medical admissions)
Fax: 0114 271 3960
Email: medadmissions@sheffield.ac.uk
Web: http://www.sheffield.ac.uk

Additional application information

Average A-level requirements	• ABB (AB in two sciences, one of which must be chemistry)
Average Scottish Higher requirements	• AAAAB + Advanced Highers at grades AB in chemistry and another science subject
Graduate entry requirements	• 2:1 science based degree + BCC at A-level
Make-up of interview panel	• Medically qualified member of staff, biomedical scientist, medical student
Months in which interviews are held	• Mid-November to mid-March
Proportion of overseas students	• 6%
Proportion of mature students	• 18.5%
Proportion of graduate students	• 14%
Faculty's view of students taking a gap year	• Acceptable
Proportion of students taking intercalated degrees	• 10%
Possibility of direct entrance to clinical phase	• Yes if places available
Fees for overseas students	• £10 200 (preclinical) £18 850 (clinical)
Fees for graduates	• £1125
Ability to transfer to other medical schools	• Yes. If the other medical school consents
Assistance for elective funding	• Adequate if apply to enough sources
Assistance for travel to attachments	• No – responsibility of LEA/ELB/SAAS
Access and hardship funds	• Available but highly selective
Weekly rent	• £50–£60
Pint of lager	• £1.50
Cinema	• £3.50
Nightclub	• Average week £3.50, average weekend £6 plus

Southampton

Key facts	Undergraduate	Graduate
Course length	5 years	4 years
Total number of medical undergraduates	975	Commencing October 2004
Applicants in 2003	2197	N/A
Interviews given in 2003	Only mature and overseas applicants are interviewed	N/A
Places available in 2003	200	N/A
Places available in 2004	200	40
Open days 2004	April, May, July, August, September	
Entrance requirements	AAB (in fourth AS-level)	2:1 degree in any discipline
Mandatory subjects	A-level chemistry or AS-level chemistry plus AS-level biology/ human biology	None
Male:female ratio	39:61	Not known yet
Is an exam included in the selection process? If yes, what form does this exam take?	No	No
Qualification gained	BM	

The medical school at Southampton University is modern and student friendly. Southampton pioneered the new integrated curriculum now in operation in most UK medical schools. As such, it has had more experience than most schools at settling in to the new ways of learning medicine. An innovative programme of multidisciplinary learning has been developed in conjunction with the School of Nursing and Midwifery, the School of Health Professions and Rehabilitation Sciences, and the University of Portsmouth. Southampton has just about everything city life has to offer, but on a scale that is easy to cope with, and, of course, it's by the sea!

Education

The fully integrated course has an increasing clinical component throughout the 5 years. During the first 2 years, each term deals with the basic science and clinical aspects of a major organ system, and includes clinical sessions in hospitals and general practice and in the labour ward. During year 3, students work in the Southampton area. Exams at the end of this year integrate basic science and clinical knowledge, a feature that is valued by students. Year 4 comprises clinical experience in the minor specialties, plus a research project. This educational innovation enables students to study an area of their choice for 8 months, finishing with a dissertation and presentation. Some are fascinated by their project, but others are not and feel they forget a lot of the first 3 years' teaching. Final-year students are spread throughout the Wessex, Surrey, and Sussex regions in large teaching hospitals and smaller district general hospitals. Southampton has complied with GMC recommendations to limit the amount of factual knowledge that is required, and as a result the examinations are not structured to make you regurgitate thousands of facts but to test your ability to solve clinical problems, that is, to be a good doctor!

Teaching

In the early years, students spend most of their time on the main university campus with other, non-medical, students learning in lectures, tutorials, and laboratory practicals as well as in general practice and in the main teaching hospital during the "medicine in practice" course. Southampton has also been introducing computer-based learning into the curriculum.

Assessment

The major exams are at the end of years 1 and 3 and throughout the final year.

Intercalated degrees

Between 5% and 15% of students take the opportunity to spend an extra year between years 3 and 4 to study for a BSc in basic or social sciences. Only a few students do this, because of the extra expense, and because all students spend time in research during year 4. From 2004, students who already have a degree can apply for the 4-year graduate entry programme.

Special study modules and electives

At the end of year 3 students have an 8-week elective during which they may decide to spend time working in a hospital abroad. There are special study modules during year 3, where students may choose to study a particular area in depth. Students undertake one unit during their medical and surgical blocks. Students have completely free choice of units, subject to availability. In year 5 there is a 5-week block when students choose which specialty to gain additional experience in.

Facilities

Library Students have access to the Biomedical Sciences Library on the main campus and the Health Sciences Library at the General Hospital. Library facilities are good, although the most popular books are always in demand and students find it more convenient to buy core texts.

Computers   The computer facilities are very good and are updated regularly. Workstations are available all over the campus, at the General Hospital, and in some halls of residence.

Clinical skills   This is an excellent facility and used in the medicine in practice course in years 1 and 2, as well as in some of the clinical attachments in years 3 and 4, and for revision during final year.

Welfare

Student support

Most people are struck by the friendliness of the staff and students at the medical school when they visit. A scheme has recently been set up whereby students run minitutorials for newer students in order to pass on the most relevant information: which books to buy, books not to buy, consultants with nice yachts who often need crew on trips round the Channel Isles – all the really important stuff. Southampton University has a counselling service, and the Students' Union has welfare services.

Accommodation

Students will be offered a place in halls of residence for their first year only. There is a range of options, from a small self-catering room with no sink, to a large en-suite room with breakfast and evening meal. The accommodation you choose though is governed by the size of your bank balance! A limited number of places are available in halls for subsequent years, but most people move into private rented houses in the Highfield and Portswood areas. Most halls are within a mile of the medical school.

Placements

The main university campus is in the Highfield/Bassett area of Southampton and is close to most of the halls of residence. The General Hospital, where most of years 3 and 4 as well as one or two days a week in years 1 and 2 are spent, is about 1 mile away in Shirley. There is a reliable university bus service connecting all sites.

Clinical attachments may be in local Southampton hospitals or, in the final year, in several hospitals in the region as far afield as Guildford or Poole. In these final-year placements there are fewer students per hospital and, consequently, more individual attention; students give excellent feedback from these placements. Accommodation and travel expenses are provided on peripheral attachments. A car is always useful but it is not necessary because every group has at least one student who is a car owner and its loads of fun to travel together!

Sports and social 🏆

City life

Southampton has been widely rebuilt, having been heavily bombed during the war. There is a wide range of shops and restaurants, and most of the amenities you would expect of a city are evident.

Location of clinical placement/name of hospital	Distance away from medical school (miles)	Difficulty getting there on public transport*
Portsmouth	24	+
Basingstoke	35	+
Bournemouth	45	++
Poole	40	++
Guildford	50	+++

*Ease of accessibility: +, set your alarm clock early; ++, long journey; +++, car is a must

There are over 35 000 students in the city, which has a range of clubs, pubs, cinemas, and eateries. The New Forest is popular for nature lovers, cyclists and "pub-lunchers", and the Solent and the Isle of Wight are popular with sailors. The proximity to Bournemouth beach is a bonus for sun and sand lovers. London is close enough for a day or night out by car, coach, or train.

University life

The Students' Union runs every club you could ever imagine wanting to join, and quite a few others besides! The Union building hosts nightclub events and bands. The on-site theatre and concert hall host lots of non-mainstream acts and performances. The medical school is renowned for its strong social life, and has a number of sporting and other societies. There is an annual ball, which is the most popular in the university, and an extravagant Christmas revue, which never fails to entertain.

Sports life

The University of Southampton has excellent water sports teams. The facilities are accessible to everyone, from those who have never sailed/rowed/canoed in their lives to those who wish to compete at an international level. Southampton has teams in most sports.

Fascinating fact: The well-organised medical society caters for all student needs and the university has its own nightclub!

Great things about Southampton

- Excellent course, well liked by students.
- Good patient/doctor:student ratio on attachments.
- Students are part of the main university, not just the medical school.
- All staff are very student friendly and approachable and there is a great support network for any problems.
- It's on the south coast so it is warm in Southampton – and it's by the sea!

Bad things about Southampton

- As it's one of the newer medical schools, some of the older consultants tend to be sceptical about any "newfangled" ways of doing things.
- Too many distractions – university social life, medical school social life, good lectures, beautiful countryside.
- The city's nightlife isn't what it could be.
- Having the elective after just one year of clinical work makes you less useful in a hospital abroad.
- Some of the fifth-year attachments can leave you feeling isolated and away from Southampton (for example, Isle of Wight), but this doesn't last too long – maximum 8 weeks.

Further information

School of Medicine Admissions Office
University of Southampton
Boldrewood Campus
Bassett Crescent East
Southampton SO16 7PX
Tel: 02380 594 408
Fax: 02380 594 159
Email: prospenq@soton.ac.uk
Bmadmissions@soton.ac.uk
Web: http://www.som.soton.ac.uk/

Additional application information

Average A-level requirements	• AAB including chemistry. AS: passes in chemistry and biology/human biology. GCSE at grade C in English, maths, and double award science (or equivalent)
Average Scottish Higher requirements	• Please check with school
Graduate entry requirements	• 2:1 degree in any discipline
Make-up of interview panel	• Academic, clinician, lay person
Months in which interviews are held	• November–March
Proportion of overseas students	• 12% per intake
Proportion of mature students	• 25% per intake
Proportion of graduate students	• 44 out of 200 total intake
Faculty's view of students taking a gap year	• Encouraged if used constructively
Proportion of students taking intercalated degrees	• 15%
Possibility of direct entrance to clinical phase	• No
Fees for overseas students	• £10 500 pa (preclinical); £19 160 pa (clinical)
Fees for graduates	• £1125
Ability to transfer to other medical schools	• If the other medical school consents
Assistance for elective funding	• None
Assistance for travel to attachments	• Some
Access and hardship funds	• Through the central university
Weekly rent	• Halls £48–£93; private £50
Pint of lager	• £1.40 union bar; £2 city pub
Cinema	• £2–£5
Nightclub	• Free–£8

Warwick

Key facts	Graduate course
Course length	4 years
Total number of medical undergraduates	480
Applicants in 2003	1000
Interviews given in 2003	500
Places available in 2003	164
Places available in 2004	164
Open days 2004	February (further dates to be confirmed)
Entrance requirements	2:1 degree
Mandatory subjects	Biological sciences
Male:female ratio	40:60
Is an exam included in the selection process? If yes, what form does this exam take?	No
Qualification gained	MBChB

The Universities of Leicester and Warwick joined in 2000 to offer an accelerated 4-year medical degree course to graduates in biomedical sciences. The course started with 64 students and the first intake began their studies at Warwick on an accelerated version of Phase I of the Leicester 5-year degree programme. Upon successful completion of Phase I, students enter the Phase II programme in the Coventry area. Warwick Medical School was formally established as a department at the University of Warwick on 1 January 2003.

Education

The curriculum is intended for biological science graduates and it is assumed you have sound knowledge of biochemistry, genetics, molecular biology, cell biology, and research methods. The course does not presume much study of the social sciences.

Students on the 4-year graduate-entry course complete Phase I (preclinical) at Warwick. Phase I is modular and lasts for three semesters. Modules cover mechanisms of disease, health policy issues, and understanding the skills and knowledge needed to be a doctor. Team working is emphasised.

There is clinical content during this phase and body systems are studied in an integrated way (studying anatomy, biochemistry, physiology, etc all at the same time).

Teaching

During Phase I students travel to Leicester for anatomy sessions (not really a placement). Hospitals and general practices used during Phase I and Phase II (clinical) are all in and around the Coventry area.

Assessment

During Phase I students on the four-year course are assessed in a way that allows for quality assurance with the 5-year course. This includes MCQ and short-answer questions.

Intercalated degrees

All students are graduates and intercalated degrees are not offered.

Special study modules and electives

There is one SSM within Phase I of the Warwick course, and one in Phase II.

Erasmus

Exchanges are not possible due to the short length of Phase I. Travel is possible during elective in Phase II.

Facilities

Library   Warwick has a huge library on the central campus. This is generally well resourced, but time will be needed to build up the core of medical knowledge to more satisfactory levels.

Computers   There are modern facilities at the medical school and no shortage of computer rooms and clusters around the campus.

Clinical skills   Several clinical rooms allow practice of basic clinical skills at the medical school. One half day per week is spent practising clinical skills in Phase I; this is in local hospitals from semester 2.

Welfare

Student support

Students can access the main university counselling and welfare services, as well as those available through the Students' Union. A personal tutor scheme operates in the school and interyear relations are good, so there is always someone you can ask advice from about the course.

Location of clinical placement/name of hospital	Distance away from medical school (miles)	Difficulty getting there on public transport*	Accommodation available
Walsgrave	5	+	No
Coventry and Warwick	3	+	No
George Elliot (Nuneaton)	20	++	Yes
Warwick	8	++	No
Alexandra (Redditch)	30	+++	Yes

*Ease of accessibility: +, set your alarm clock early; ++, long journey; +++, car is a must

Accommodation

Accommodation in university halls is not guaranteed for 1 year. However, prospective first-year students are accommodated in nearby university flats in Earlsdon, Canley, and Coventry. Non-medics living out in private accommodation stay mainly in Leamington Spa or one of the areas of Coventry adjacent to the university (Earlsdon, Canley), a bus or car ride away from the campus.

Placements

The medical school building is at Gibbet Hill, a quiet part of the campus, a short walk away from the main centre. The brand new buildings are excellent and well equipped (although there are some concerns about a shortage of space already). Students have a common room with pigeon holes, some catering facilities, and a balcony available to them. The main teaching hospitals are George Elliot (Nuneaton), Walsgrave, Warwick Hospital, and the Coventry and Warwick Hospital.

Sports and social 🏆

City life

Warwick might have been named Coventry University when it was founded. It may be in Warwickshire, but it is really a part of Coventry. Coventry suffered terribly in the Blitz and much of the centre was unimaginatively rebuilt. One notable exception is the new cathedral, which was built within the remains of the old one. It does, however, have almost everything you might expect of a medium-sized city: theatre, museums, good shopping, restaurants, and travel links. It was the centre of the British car industry and retains Jaguar, Land Rover, and Peugeot plants. Coventry cannot boast the success of Leicester in terms of national sporting prowess, as both its rugby and football teams are no longer Premiership quality.

A short journey in any direction can get you into pretty countryside, and places to visit in Warwickshire include Kenilworth Castle, Warwick and Warwick Castle, and Stratford-upon-Avon.

University life

In spite of its relative youth, Warwick has a busy MedSoc, which runs regular events for medics. The inaugural student-run freshers' week was a success, with pub crawls, a toga party, and a bowling night being hits with the new students. Students at Warwick can take advantage of a wide range of facilities on campus. A large Students' Union provides a wide range of entertainment: bands, balls, and student theatre are all regular events. A large and busy Arts Centre hosts many touring theatre and dance companies, as well as music of all types. Banks, shops, and a post office are all on the doorstep.

Sports life

There are many sports facilities at Warwick, including an athletics track, swimming pool, playing fields, and sports centre. All the main sports are catered for, as well as many less popular ones.

Fascinating fact: Warwick medical school was the first graduate entry course to admit science graduates.

Great things about Warwick 👍

- Brand new building with a state-of-the-art lecture theatre.
- Great Arts Centre on campus.
- Significant clinical content from early on in the course and clinical application of what is learnt is constantly emphasised.
- State-of-the-art video equipment beams teaching to us from anywhere in the world – but mainly from Leicester!
- There is some excitement about being part of a new way of doing things.

Bad things about Warwick 👎

- Travelling to Leicester for part of the course is time consuming.
- Some of the organisation and timetabling has not been sympathetic to students.
- At the end of a long day it is often a tiring journey home if you live off-campus.
- Car parking during the day on campus is expensive, and you sometimes feel as if Warwick University exists purely to make money.
- Some of the student accommodation areas are quite a distance from Phase II District General Hospitals.

Further information

Undergraduate Admissions Team
University of Warwick
Gibbet Hill Campus
Coventry
CV4 7AL
Tel: 02476 528 101/574 550 (medical admissions)
     02476 523 723 (undergraduate admissions)
Fax: 02476 524 586
Email: med-admis@warwick.ac.uk
Web: http://www.lwms.ac.uk

Additional application information

Average A-level requirements	• N/A
Average Scottish Higher requirements	• N/A
Graduates entry requirements	• 2:1 degree in biological sciences
Make-up of interview panel	• One senior doctor plus one other (from senior student, non-clinical academic, health professional)
Months in which interviews are held	• November–March
Proportion of overseas students	• 3.5%
Proportion of mature students	• 100%
Proportion of graduate students	• 100%
Faculty's view of students taking a gap year	• Acceptable
Proportion of students taking intercalated degrees	• 0%
Possibility of direct entrance to clinical phase	• No
Fees for overseas students	• £9900 (year 1); £18 825 (years 2, 3, 4)
Fees for graduates	• See Chapter 6
Ability to transfer to other medical schools	• Contact admissions directly for information
Assistance for elective funding	• Contact admissions directly for information
Assistance for travel to attachments	• None
Access and hardship funds	• Available
Weekly rent	• £45–£55 halls; £55 private
Pint of lager	• £1.20 Union bar; £1.70 city pub
Cinema	• £2.80 with NUS card
Nightclub	• Free–£10

Appendices

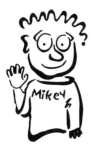

Mikey's quick compare table

Mikey's quick compare table

University	No. applicants (2003)	No. places (2003)	% interviewed	Entrance req.	Manditory subject	M:F	% Intercalated year	% mature	% overseas	Graduate course
Aberdeen	1310	185	77	ABB	Chemistry	39/61	20	27	8	No
Barts	2000	268	56	ABB	Chemistry and biology	116:155	60	25	9	Yes
Belfast	595	180	4	AAA + a in AS	Chemistry and biology	39/61	10	3	7	No
Birmingham	1614	346	68	AAB	Chemistry and biology	02:03	20	6	7.62	Yes
Brighton & Sussex	1000	128	50	ABB	Chemistry and biology	42:58	0 at present	28	0	No
Bristol	1852	217	37	AAB	Chemistry + other science	01:02	30	6	5	Yes
Cambridge	1190	278	99	AAA	Chemistry	46:54	100	5	7	Yes
Cardiff	1459	298	55	ABB	Chemistry and biology	33:67	20	11	7	Yes
Dundee	1169	154	47	AAB	Chemistry	43:57	6	3	7.5	No
East Anglia	900	110	50	AAB	Biology	40:60	0 at present	No info	0	No
Edinburgh	2050	218	2	AAAB	Chemistry and biology	35:65	40	5	7.5	No
Glasgow	1321	241	64	AAB	Chemistry	36:64	30		7.5	No
GKT	3300	360	36	ABB/C	Chemistry and biology	35:64	50	16	7.5	Yes
Hull & York	1100	130	71	AAB	Chemistry and biology	3.5:6.5	0 at present	20	0	No
Imperial	2315	326	39	ABB + A in AS	Chemistry and biology	44:56	100	2.5	7	No
Leeds	2105	223	37	AAB	Chemistry	37:63	40	5	6	No

(Continued)

Mikey's quick compare table (continued)

University	No. applicants (2003)	No. places (2003)	% interviewed	Entrance req.	Mandatory subject	M:F	% Intercalated year	% mature	% overseas	Graduate course
Leicester	1500	175	53	AAA	Chemistry and biology	60:40	10	10	8	Yes
Liverpool	1672	281	60	AAA	Chemistry and biology	40:60	10	3	7.5	Yes
Manchester/ Keele/Preston	2333	341	46	AAB	Chemistry	44:56	5	10	6	No
Newcastle/ Durham	2500	315	33	AAB	Chemistry and/or biology	60:40	9	10	6	Yes
Nottingham/ Derby	2400	245	37.5	AAB	Chemistry and biology	40:60	All students do a BMedSci without doing an extra year	10	10	Yes
Oxford	941	150	87	AAA	Chemistry	45:55	100	2	5	Yes
Peninsula	1027	167	74	AAA + 1AS	One science		0 at present	20	0	No
Royal Free & UCL	2340	330	42	AAB + 1AS	Chemistry and biology	02:03	100	No info	8	No
St Andrew's	557	125	9	ABB	Chemistry + other science	40:60	10	4	20	No
St George's	1600	187	44	ABB + b in AS	Chemistry and biology	02:03	25	30	7·5	Yes
Sheffield	2600	238	37	ABB	Chemistry + other science	1:1.7	10	18.5	6	No
Southampton	2197	200	mature & o/s only	AAB	Chemistry	39:61	15	25	12	Yes
Warwick	1000	164	50	2:1 degree	Biological sciences	40:60	0	100	3.5	Yes

Glossary

Medicine is full of jargon and abbreviations. Estimates suggest that students' vocabularies double over the course of a 5-year medical degree. Unfortunately, it is such a part of life for medical students and doctors that they sometimes forget to speak in plain language to the general public. The following is a very brief list of words pertaining to medical education that you are likely to come across in this guide, and perhaps in medical school prospectuses. Our apologies for any jargon we have used in the guide not listed here!

Anatomy: The study of the structure of the body. Whilst this used to be taught by dissection, prosections (predissected specimens) are more commonly used nowadays.

Attachment: The term given to clinical placements. The student is placed under the supervision and guidance of a hospital consultant and his/her team (firm) or a GP for a period in the course.

Biochemistry: The study of the structure and functioning of the body at the molecular level.

British Medical Association (BMA): The doctors' professional association and trade union, providing representation and services for doctors and medical students.

BSc (Honours): *see* Intercalated degrees.

Clerking: Taking a history from and examining a patient on admission. A very useful learning experience if you are the first person to see the patient.

Computer-assisted learning (CAL): Computer programs are sometimes used to teach a topic in a more interactive format than a lecture/tutorial, and let the student set his/her own learning pace. They may also give the opportunity for self-assessment on a topic.

Consultant: The senior specialist doctor, usually based in a hospital.

Core curriculum: Under GMC directives the medical course is split into a core curriculum (in which all students must cover the same key topics to a high standard) and special study modules (in which the student can go in his/her own direction and study an area of interest in more depth), which may not be covered by all students.

District general hospital (DGH): A regional hospital that treats a broad spectrum of patients but refers more specialist cases to a teaching hospital. Medical students are taught by NHS staff, not university-employed consultants and registrars.

Elective: A period (usually 6–12 weeks in the latter years of the course) when students can choose an area of interest to study independently outside their medical school, either in the UK or, more often, abroad.

Endocrinology: The study of the hormonal function of the body.

Epidemiology: The study of the pattern and causes of diseases in society.

Firm: *see* Attachment.

Foundation Programme: New programme of two-year posts taken up immediately after graduation from medical school, to be introduced in 2005 for all UK graduates.

General Medical Council (GMC): All medical degree courses must be approved by the GMC. It is the medical profession's self-regulatory body, which ensures professional standards are maintained and patients are protected. Doctors must be registered with the GMC to practise in the UK.

Honours year: *see* Intercalated degrees.

Integrated courses: Integration is the merging of several disciplines into one (hopefully more meaningful) course. Integration may be partial, within a single year or Phase (for example combining anatomy, physiology, and biochemistry to teach body systems – respiratory, cardiovascular, reproduction etc), or it may be full, across all years, starting clinical teaching with basic medical sciences from the outset.

Intercalated degrees: Most schools offer students the opportunity to take an extra year (or two) in the middle of the course to study a subject of interest, leading to a BSc (Hons) or equivalent at the end. Some schools only offer this to high achievers, while others have an intercalated BSc (Hons) built into the course for everyone.

MBBS: The degree awarded to medical school graduates. (This varies slightly between schools, for example MBChB, MBBChir, but all are equivalent.)

Medical microbiology: The study of micro-organisms and the diseases they cause.

Medical Students Committee (BMA): UK committee of elected representatives that looks after the interests of all UK medical students.

MedLine: A widely used and comprehensive computer database of articles published in medical journals.

Objective Structured Clinical Examination (OSCE): A relatively new form of assessment where the students are set several tasks: taking histories; examining patients; or performing tests/ procedures to complete in front of the examiner within a set time. The student is marked according to a standardised marking scheme. Every student is thus assessed identically, ensuring fairness and comparability of results between individuals.

Pathology: The study of disease processes and their effect on the structure and function of the body.

Peripheral attachments: Placements in hospitals/general practices outside the university area and normally outside the university town.

Pharmacology: The study of the action of drugs and their application.

Physiology: The study of the functioning of body systems and tissues.

Premedical year: Students without the necessary science entrance qualifications can apply to do a premedical year, which takes them to a sufficient level of scientific knowledge to join the medical course the following academic year (not offered at all schools).

Preregistration house officer (PRHO): A newly qualified doctor working in the first year after graduation. House officers, while able to call themselves doctors and prescribe drugs, are provisionally registered by the GMC until they have completed this year satisfactorily. After this they achieve full registration.

Problem-based learning (PBL): Students learn from researching and solving a relevant (usually clinical) scenario, rather than being given all the information passively. Small-group problem-solving tutorials, facilitated by members of staff, take the place of lectures.

Prosections: Predissected cadaver specimens of the human body used to teach anatomy. These have replaced actual dissection by students themselves in many schools.

Provisional Registration: Conditional registration with the GMC after graduation from medical school. Full registration is granted at the end of the first year of working once competencies are achieved.

Registrar: A doctor who is undergoing specialist training (usually for between 3 and 9 years) before becoming a consultant or general practitioner. The next step up the ladder after SHO.

Self-directed learning: Learning under the student's own initiative from lists of objectives rather than didactic teaching (such as lectures).

Senior house officer (SHO): A junior hospital doctor who has completed his/her year as house officer.

Special study modules (SSMs): Periods of the course when students study areas of interest outside the core curriculum (see above). These may be taught, or may be independent research projects.

Teaching hospitals: Normally the main hospital(s) in the university town or city. Services provided are part of the NHS, but the senior clinical staff will often be employed by the university and hold medical academic posts. Teaching hospitals usually handle specialist cases, which can be referred to them from DGHs across the region. Many such hospitals will have regional centres for particular specialties or centres of excellence, such as cardiology, plastic surgery, neonatal intensive care etc.

Viva: An oral examination (sometimes referred to as a viva voce).

Abbreviations

BMA:	British Medical Association
BMAT:	Biomedical admissions test
CAL:	Computer-assisted learning
CSYS:	Certificate of sixth-year study (Scottish students)
DGH:	District general hospital
GMC:	General Medical Council
MCQs:	Multiple choice questionnaires
MSC:	BMA's UK Medical Students Committee
OSCE:	Objective structured clinical examination
PBL:	Problem-based learning
PRHO:	Preregistration house officer
SHO:	Senior house officer
SSM:	Special study module
UCAS:	Universities and Colleges Admissions Service

Further information

British Medical Association

The British Medical Association (BMA) is both the doctors' professional organisation and their trade union, protecting the professional and personal interests of its members. It is the voice of the medical profession in the UK and represents the profession internationally. Members and staff are in constant touch with ministers, government departments, Members of Parliament, and other influential bodies, conveying to them the profession's views on health care and health policy. Most medical students and practising doctors are members.

The BMA's head office is in London, and there are national offices in Scotland, Northern Ireland, and Wales. There are an additional 15 regional offices throughout the UK. The BMA is a medical publisher in its own right, but also includes the BMJ Publishing Group. The BMJ Publishing Group is a major medical and scientific publisher and publishes the weekly *British Medical Journal* and the monthly *Student BMJ*.

Student BMJ   The *Student BMJ* is an international journal specifically for medical students. It is published monthly and includes articles on education, medical careers, student life, science, and news. Many of the articles and papers are written by medical students. Individuals or schools and libraries can subscribe to the journal.

For more information or a sample copy contact:

Student BMJ
BMJ Publishing Group
BMA House
Tavistock Square
London WC1H 9JR

Tel: 020 7383 6402
Fax: 020 7383 6270
Email: bmjsubs@dial.pipex.com
Web: http://www.studentbmj.com

BMA Medical Students Committee (MSC)

The Medical Students Committee (MSC) represents students within the Association and also to important outside bodies, such as the Departments of Education and Health and the General Medical Council. Through the committee the BMA campaigns on many issues, such as student finances and debt, reforms of the medical degree syllabus, and health and safety. Following devolution the BMA has established MSCs in Northern Ireland, Scotland, and Wales. There are student representatives and BMA committees in every medical school, and the BMA runs many local events and talks for students. The majority of medical students join the BMA.

Medical students who are members of the BMA receive a variety of benefits, including a free subscription to *Student BMJ*, free guidance notes, a free copy of *Clinical Evidence*, library and information services, and book discounts to name but a few. General information, guidance, and a student chat board can be found on the BMA's Medical Students Committee website. For more information contact:

British Medical Association
BMA House
Tavistock Square
London WC1H 9JP

Tel: 020 7387 4499
Fax: 020 7383 6494
Email: students@bma.org.uk
Web: http://www.bma.org.uk/students

The rest of this chapter is divided into sections relating to education, finance, and welfare corresponding to the different subcommittees within the MSC. Information in the cooperative members section relates to other medical student organisations that have a member that sits on the MSC.

Education

Universities and Colleges Admissions Service (UCAS)

Universities and Colleges
Admissions Service
Rose Hill
New Barn Lane
Cheltenham
Gloucestershire GL52 3LZ

Tel: 01242 222444
Web: http://www.ucas.com

- *UCAS Handbook and Application Pack*: essential reading and material for applicants to university courses.

Department for Education and Skills

The Scottish Office
Web: http://www.dfes.gov.uk/studentsupport

There are many publications about higher education and funding for Scottish students available on the web or from:

The Stationery Office
Lothian Road
Edinburgh EH3 9AZ

Tel: 0131 228 4181 71
Fax: 0131 622 7017
Web: http://www.scotland.gov.uk

Financial information

Financial arrangements and support vary depending on which country you live in and which country you intend studying in. Some support is provided by Departments of Education and Skills, and some from Departments of Health.

The Educational Grants Advisory Service provides information about student support systems in the UK and can help identify additional sources of funding.

Family Welfare Association
501–505 Kingsland Road
London E8 4AU

Tel: 0207 254 6251 (opening hours: Mondays,
    Wednesdays, and Fridays 10 am–12 pm, and 2 pm–4 pm)
Email: egas.enquiry@fwa.org.uk
Web: http://www.egas-online.org.uk

Relevant contact information for each nation is below.

England

For information and guides on student support ring the Department for Education and Skills (DFES):

Helpline: 0800 731 9133
Web: http://www.dfes.gov.uk

- *Financial Help for Health Care Students*, a booklet by the Department of Health, explains NHS funding in more detail. Order one or download from the website:

Department of Health
PO Box 777
London SE1 6XH

Tel: 0845 60 60 655
Email: doh@prologistics.co.uk
Web: http://www.doh.gov.uk/hcsmain.htm

You can obtain bursary information from:

NHS Student Grants Unit
22 Plymouth Road
Blackpool FY3 7JS

Tel: 01253 655655
Fax: 01253 206 1499
Email: nhs-sgu@ukonline.co.uk

Scotland

Student Awards Agency for Scotland
3 Redheughs Rigg
South Gyle
Edinburgh EH12 9YT

Tel: 0131 476 8227
Web: http://www.student-support-saas.gov.uk/

Wales

Further and Higher Education Division of the National Assembly for Wales
Tel: 02920 825 831
Web: http://www.learning.wales.gov.uk

You can obtain bursary information from:

NHS Wales Student Awards Unit
2nd Floor Golate House
101 St Mary's St
Cardiff CF10 1DX
Tel: 02920 261 495

Northern Ireland

Information for students from Northern Ireland can be obtained from the Department for Employment and Learning:

Web: http://www.delni.gov.uk

Also try:

The Department of Health   Tel: 02890 524746
Social Services and Public Safety Web: http://www.dhsspsni.gov.uk
Human Resources Directorate

Charities

Copies of the following books should be available in the reference section of most public libraries:

- *The Charities Digest* – published by the Family Welfare Association
- *Money to Study* – published by UKOSA/NUS/EGAS
- *The Educational Grants Directory* – published by the Directory of Social Change
- *Directory of Grant-Making Trusts* – published by Charities Aid Foundation/Biblios.

The British Medical Association Charities Office (see BMA address) has information about awards and grants for mature and second degree medical students.

Welfare

National Union of Students (NUS)

For general information on issues relating to students:

National Union of Students Tel: 020 7272 8900
Nelson Mandela House   Fax: 020 7263 5713
Holloway Road   Email: nusuk@nus.org.uk
London N7 6LJ   Web: http://www.nusonline.co.uk

Gay and Lesbian Association of Doctors and Dentists (GLADD)

GLADD was formed in 1995. It has an active student section and provides professional support, educational and social meetings, both locally and nationally. GLADD campaigns vigorously within the health service and in the country at large on issues of equality relating to the lesbian, gay, and bisexual community.

Email: gladd@dircon.co.uk
Web: http://www.gladd.dircon.co.uk

Skill

National Bureau for Students with Disabilities is a registered, national charity, which promotes opportunities for disabled people in further and higher education, training, and employment. Skill operates a freephone information service that provides expert information on studying and training – from applying to university or college through to obtaining a Disabled Students Allowance and getting adjustments in exams. Skill also works with policy-makers, tutors, and disabled student advisers to ensure that disabled students are empowered to achieve their potential.

Information Service
Tel: 0800 328 5050 (voice)/0800 068 2422 (text)
Email: info@skill.org.uk
Web: www.skill.org.uk

Other organisations

Christian Medical Fellowship (CMF)

CMF has over 5500 medical student and doctor members throughout the UK and Ireland. It exists to encourage fellowship, Christian ethics, evangelism, and medical mission, and to provide a Christian voice on medical issues. CMF runs conferences, coordinates local groups, and publishes widely at the interface of Christianity and medicine. It is one of 60 member bodies of the International Christian Medical and Dental Association (ICMDA). A publications catalogue and information about local groups, conferences, and activities are available from:

Dr Mark Pickering
Student Secretary
Christian Medical Fellowship
157 Waterloo Road
London SE1 8XN

Tel: 020 7928 4694
Fax: 020 7620 2453
Email: student@cmf.org.uk or admin@cmf.org.uk
Web: http://www.cmf.org.uk

Medical Students International Network (MedSIN)

Founded in 1997, MedSIN is an independent, student-run organisation that aims to facilitate medical students' involvement in humanitarian and educational activities at local, national, and international level. MedSIN groups in medical schools carry out sex education projects, international exchanges, bone marrow registration drives, seminars on topical issues, and much more. Through its membership of the International Federation of Medical Students' Associations (IFMSA), MedSIN also provides opportunities to help on projects all over the world, from Angola to Zimbabwe. The IFMSA was founded in 1951 and promotes international cooperation on professional training and the achievement of humanitarian ideals. To get in touch or find out more, visit the MedSIN website: http://www.medsin.org

Other useful information

Armed forces: cadet recruitment

Army

Royal Army Medical Corps
Recruiting Office
Regimental Headquarters
Army Medical Services
Slim Road
Camberley GU14 4NP

Tel: 01276 412730
Fax: 01276 412731
Email: ramc.recruiting@army.mod.uk.net

RAF

Medical and Dental Liaison Officer
Directorate of Recruiting and Selection
(Royal Air Force)
PO Box 100
Cranwell
Sleaford NG34 8GZ

Tel: 01400 261201 ext 6811
Fax: 01400 262220
Email: mdlo@royalairforce.net

Royal Navy

Med Pers (N)2
Room 133
Victory Building
HM Naval Base
Portsmouth PO1 3LS

Tel: 02392 727818
Fax: 02392 727805

Further reading

- *Learning Medicine* by Peter Richards (formerly Dean of St Mary's Medical School) and Simon Stockill, published by BMJ Publishing Group and updated regularly. Now in its

16th edition, this title is available from the BMJ Bookshop. Price £13.95 (discount available for BMA members). Tel: 020 7383 6244. Web: http://www.bmjbookshop.com.
- *Medical Careers: a General Guide* (3rd revised edition): this publication is available free of charge to BMA members from their local BMA office, or at £10 to non-members from the BMJ Bookshop. Tel: 020 7383 6244. General information on getting into medical schools is available from the BMA website.

Mind Readings